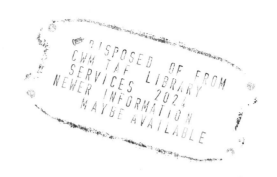

Published by Wolfe Medical Publications Ltd,
London, England
Printed by Smeets-Weert, Holland
ISBN 0 7234 0724 X

To our wives

Anne & Talya

Acknowledgements

This six-volume colour atlas of Gynaecological Surgery was produced at the Jessop Hospital for Women, Sheffield as part of a postgraduate project to teach operative surgery by edited colour slides. We are indebted to all who took part in the exercise, but there are some whom we would particularly like to mention.

Mr Alan Tunstill, Head, Department of Medical Illustration, Sheffield Area Health Authority (Teaching), organised the whole of the actual photography. Mr Stephen Hirst took nearly all the photographs; the high standard of his work is obvious.

Professor I. D. Cooke generously gave full access to clinical material in his unit. Mr David Millar and Mr Miles Fox kindly allowed us to photograph the first case in Chapter 13.

The anaesthetists at all levels were very co-operative. Dr A. G. D. Nicholas, Dr D. R. Powell and Professor J. A. Thornton were the consultants involved. Of the numerous senior registrars we remember particularly Drs Bailey, Birks, Burt, Clark, Dye, Mullins, Saunders and Stacey.

Miss J. Hughes-Nurse, Mr I. V. Scott, Miss P. Buck and Dr H. David were the senior registrars and lecturers in obstetrics and gynaecology during the time and greatly assisted by keeping us informed of suitable cases and in the organising of operations. Drs Katherine Jones, E. Lachman, Janet Patrick, K. Edmonds, A. Bar-am and C. Rankin were involved in the management of the cases and assisted at operations.

Miss M. Crowley, nursing officer in charge of the Jessop Hospital operating theatres saw that we had every facility, and Sisters J. Taylor, M. Henderson, E. Duffield, M. Waller and A. Broadley each acted as theatre sister or 'scrub' nurse at the individual operations. Mr Leslie Gilbert and Mr Gordon Dalton, the operating room assistants were valuable members of the team. We particularly wish to thank the whole theatre staff for their courtesy and efficiency.

Miss Sue Hunter drew some of the line drawings that appear in the text. Further line drawings and the colour diagrams are all the work of Mr Patrick Elliott, Medical Artist in the Department of Medical Illustrations, Hallamshire Hospital, Sheffield. Mr Brian Lieberman of St Mary's Hospital, London, and Dr John Marlow of Washington, United States each provided laparoscopic photographs which appear in Chapter 9.

A large amount of secretarial work was involved and we are grateful to Mrs Valerie Prior for her assistance.

Contents

Introduction

There is probably no substitute for the type of personal tuition provided by teacher and pupil working together in the operating theatre as surgeon and assistant, with knowledge and experience being passed on directly. There is, however, the disadvantage that such a relationship is not available to everyone and is, at best, transient. In addition the learner is frequently not at a stage in his career when he can take full advantage of what is available. The majority, therefore, have to look elsewhere for such instruction.

Textbooks of operative surgery provide the principal source of information, but these are only as good as their illustrations. The occasional colour plate does not instruct and there is something unreal about the well-executed drawings prepared by a medical artist to the specification of the author. The one worthwhile teaching aid is the simple line diagram or sketch, which demands considerable skill and ingenuity and allows the student to see and follow what is required. But to carry that information in one's mind and apply it in practice is another matter. In surgery, with all its accompanying distractions, the real life structures are frighteningly different from those which the simple diagrams have led one to expect, and these same structures obstinately refuse to adopt the position and behaviour expected of them.

Cine films are excellent but the cost of their production in time and money is high, besides which they are clumsy to use. This series of atlases offers what we consider to be the next best thing: a series of step-by-step colour photographs accompanied by an appropriate written commentary. This form of presentation follows almost exactly the colour slide plus commentary method most often used to teach surgery. Using slides, of course, it is necessary to have projection apparatus and access to a library or bank of suitable material. The method adopted in this series – of using high quality colour reproduction processes – retains the advantages of the slide and commentary method while avoiding its drawbacks.

The present series of atlases sets out to provide detailed instruction in the techniques of standard gynaecological operations. Its methodology is straightforward. The technique of each operation is clearly shown, step-by-step, using life-size photographs in natural colour, and with liberal use of indicators and accompanying diagrams. Where a step is repetitive or there is a natural sequence of steps, grouping has sometimes been used, but the natural size of the structures is maintained.

The accompanying commentary is concise and is printed on the same page as the photograph or photographs to which it refers. Every effort has been made to include only necessary material, but in situations where experience and special training have provided additional information and knowledge, that has been included.

The illustrations are selected and the accompanying commentaries so arranged as to carry the reader forward in a logical progression of thought and action in which he becomes involved. Occupied with one step he is at the same time anticipating the next, and in due course confirms his foresight as logical and correct. The photographs are those of a real patient having a real operation and the picture seen is exactly what the reader will see in the operation theatre when he does it himself. Interest is concentrated on the one step of the operation being taken at that time.

In any form of medical teaching there is the inevitable problem of pitching instruction at the level required by the audience and the presumption that the reader has insight into the specialist knowledge of the author is just as irritating as being patronised. We do not think there is a problem in this context because an atlas is by definition a guide and therefore for general use. It is just as likely to be consulted by a junior house surgeon about to assist at his first hysterectomy as by a senior colleague seeking an alternative method of dealing with a particular problem. That, at least, is the spirit in which it has been written.

Certain assumptions have had to be made to avoid verbosity, tediousness and sheer bulk of paper. It is hoped that the reader will be kind enough to attribute any omissions and shortcomings to the acceptance of such a policy. No one should be embarking on any of the procedures described without training in surgical principles, nor should he attempt them without knowledge of abdominal and pelvic anatomy and physiology.

Several areas have purposely been avoided in preparing the Atlas. There is no attempt to advise on the indications for operative treatment and only in the most general terms are the uses of a particular operation discussed. Individual surgeons develop their own ideas on pre- and post-operative care and have their personal predilections regarding forms of anaesthesia, fluid replacement and the use of antibiotics.

Even on the purely technical aspects the temptation to advise on the choice of instruments and surgical materials is largely resisted and it is assumed that the reader is capable of placing secure knots and ligatures. Each volume of the Atlas contains a photograph of the instruments used by the authors and some of these are shown individually. Most readers will have their own favourites but the information may be useful to younger colleagues. We do not consider the choice of suture material to be of over-riding importance. The senior author has used PGA suture material since its inception and although generally preferring it to catgut does not consider it perfect. It has disadvantages and can be very sore on the surgeon's hands but it does have advantages in that it is particularly suitable for vaginal work and for closing the abdomen.

There are, of course, several methods of performing the various operations but those described here have consistently given the authors the best results. It need hardly be reiterated that the observance of basic surgical principles is probably more important than anything else.

The Atlas is produced in six volumes, each of which relates approximately to a regional subspecialty. This is done primarily to keep the size of the volumes convenient for use but also to allow publication to proceed progressively.

From what has been written it might appear that the authors think of gynaecologists as necessarily male. The suggestion is rejected: the old-fashioned usage of the inclusive masculine gender is merely retained for simplicity and neatness. Anyone questioning the sincerity of this explanation would have to be reminded that every gynaecologist must, in the very nature of things, be a feminist.

Introduction to Volume 2

Operations for necessary inclusion in this section would demand more space than is available if the volumes were to be of uniform size. The publishers have provided some latitude in this respect, but even so there have been difficult choices about what to include and how much coverage to give each operation. In doing so the authors have tried to keep sight of what they set out to do in the first place.

The aim of the Atlas is to provide detailed instruction in the techniques of everyday standard gynaecological operations, making sure that the reader is clearly informed on one safe and precise method. This is without prejudice to other methods which in different circumstances might possibly be superior. The irreducible amount of space required is always exceeded by the policy of taking nothing for granted and insisting on repetition and revision where thought necessary. As examples of the difficult choices mentioned it could be said that appendicectomy need not be included in this volume. Sometimes, however, it is quite necessary to remove the appendix. We also believe that a gynaecological surgeon should always make an appraisal of the appendix and its condition during any pelvic operation and remove the appendix if excision is indicated. The patient may indeed already have asked the surgeon to do so in their preoperative discussion. On such considerations it was decided to include appendicectomy. The coverage given to the various conditions demanding modified hysterectomy techniques might likewise seem excessive. Again these are problems the practising gynaecological surgeon continually meets; he should not only be aware of such problems but also know how to deal with them.

In regard to laparoscopy and particularly its use for sterilisation, there is a slight departure from the policy of selecting a single method for instruction. That has been done because laparoscopy itself is still a relatively new procedure. Its use is not so widespread as one might imagine and unless the surgeon uses it frequently for purposes of sterilisation it can be dangerous. Sterilisation through the laparoscope has seen the development of many different methods and techniques with as yet no clear evidence as to which is the best and safest. In the circumstances we felt that we had to keep all the options open for the present at least.

In the Introduction to Volume 1, leaving aside personal preferences, the choice of operation for genuine stress incontinence was seen to lie between a sling procedure and a cystourethropexy. We described our cruciate sling operation which is predominantly a vaginal method in Volume 1; in this volume we have shown the Marshall–Marchetti–Krantz operation as primarily an abdominal procedure.

Regarding vesicovaginal fistula the authors firmly believe that principles are the fundamental consideration in this condition, and also believe that the general but concise diagrammatic instruction for vaginal closure in Volume 1 is appropriate. In Volume 2 we have taken into account circumstances where abdominal closure of a vesicovaginal fistula is the only suitable or possible method and also that a general surgeon doing the operation may need gynaecological guidance. The main steps in transvesical management of a large vesicovaginal fistula are illustrated and the case is taken as an instruction model. As with vaginal closure principles are paramount and are referred to in the text.

The abdominal management of a high rectovaginal fistula is included as the method usually required at high vaginal level. The more usual low rectovaginal fistulae are closed vaginorectally and the operation is demonstrated in Volume 4 of the series. As was pointed out in the Introduction to Volume 1 the Atlas classification is somewhat untidy by traditional standards. However, it is at the same time more realistic.

There is one point of anatomical nomenclature which should be mentioned. The reader will notice that in describing pelvic operations 'ovarian pedicle' is preferred to infundibulopelvic ligament although the terms are synonymous. This has been done both for neatness and to avoid the word 'ligament' which could be confusing in this context.

1: Surgical anatomy and instruments

There are two particular hazards or groups of hazards associated with pelvic surgery and each has its origins in specific anatomical factors. The first is the ease with which the ureters or the bladder can be damaged at operation; the second is the occasional occurrence of persistent and uncontrollable bleeding from deep on the side wall of the pelvis.

Bladder and ureters

The best safeguard against damage to the bladder and ureter is a concise knowledge of the anatomy of the lower renal tract and especially of the ureter. It is essential to know the exact course of the ureter in normal circumstances, its relationship to other structures and its blood supply.

The bladder is closely applied and adherent to the anterior aspect of the lower uterus and the cervix and at hysterectomy the two organs have to be separated by sharp dissection. Therefore, there is an obvious and potential hazard to the integrity of the bladder during hysterectomy. The necessary precautions are simple and will be referred to in the text.

The ureters present a greater problem. They are vulnerable over a considerable distance and at certain specific points. If divided the ureter can be very difficult to repair immediately and if injury is not recognised at the time, it causes much trouble and anxiety to both patient and surgeon.

The ureter enters the true pelvis at the level of the bifurcation of the common iliac artery. It is external and adherent to the parietal pelvic peritoneum and runs downwards and slightly medially on a converging course with numerous parallel blood vessels on the side wall of the pelvis. The ureter picks up part of its blood supply from each vessel it crosses. It is surrounded by its own areolar tissue mesentery and a closely enmeshed network of blood vessels which are fed from the vessels encountered throughout its whole length. In the iliac fossa it receives branches from the iliolumbar and the ovarian arteries and it picks up further branches from the internal pudendal and middle rectal arteries as it descends into the pelvis. In the rest of its course, and where it particularly concerns the gynaecologist, it receives contributions from the uterine, the vaginal and the middle and inferior vesical arteries. As it nears the bladder the superior and other vesical arteries send back branches along the ureter to anastomose with those from above. The concept of distinct and visible arteries running towards the ureter to furnish a blood supply is erroneous. Advice to preserve this or that vessel is confusing and dangerous because such branches will not be immediately visible and searching for them may cause tissue disturbance and bleeding. The safest approach to the ureter is to disturb it from its bed as little as ever possible and certainly refrain from stripping it of its mesentery. Otherwise the damaged blood supply may well lead to necrosis and subsequent fistula formation. This afferent blood supply is maintained intact by avoiding separation of the ureter and so preserving the mesentery. The distributive network of nutrient vessels is preserved by gentle handling, care with diathermy coagulation and avoidance of any kinking or constriction when reconstituting the pelvic peritoneum. Where it is necessary to displace the ureters laterally this can always be done without disturbing the surrounding leash of vessels. It should be remembered that the greatest danger to the ureter is the vulnerability of its own blood supply.

1

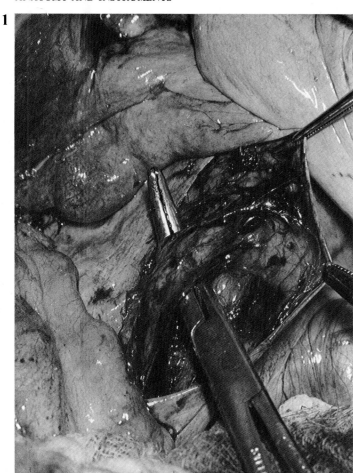

2

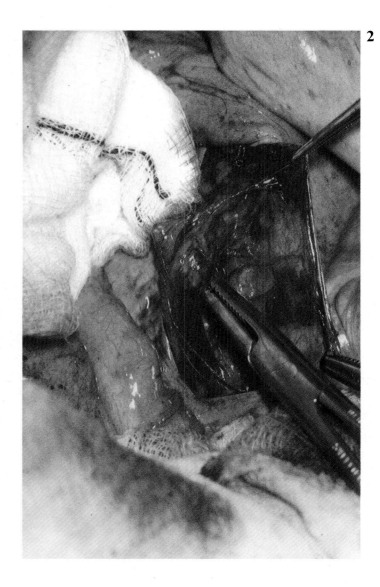

1 Exposure of ureter to show vascular network on its surface

This figure shows the enveloping network of blood vessels on the lower ureter, which contrary to accepted opinion has a very rich blood supply. The branches from the various pelvic arteries anastomose to form this continuous and tortuous chain which also has attachments to the peritoneum. At a slightly lower level than shown here the ureter is surrounded by a dense plexus of veins which communicates with the internal iliac plexus and vein. There is no lack of blood supply to the actual ureter; the problem is that it is particularly vulnerable during surgery.

2 Exposure of ureter to show its surrounding and attached mesentery

The word 'mesentery' has been used in relation to the blood supply of the lower ureter, although it is not one that will be found in anatomical textbooks. The figure shows a leash of vessels loosely surrounding the ureter and with a firm attachment deep to it to form a sub-ureteric bed. Forceps are used to elevate the ureter and the blood vessels are thrown into relief. Nearer the bladder the wall of the ureter becomes even more bound up with surrounding structures and blood supply as there is an aggregation of longitudinal muscle fibres on the surface of the muscular coat and referred to as the 'sheath of the ureter'. In view of all these anatomical considerations, it is clearly of great importance that the ureter be disturbed from its bed as little as possible and certainly never stripped of its mesentery.

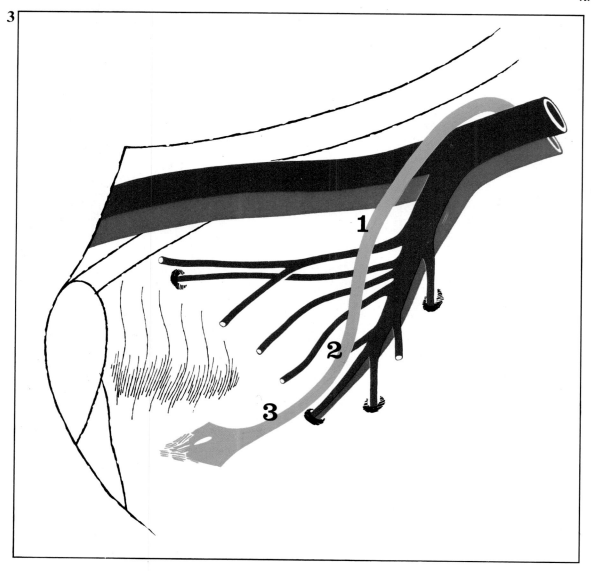

3 Relationship of ureter to blood vessels of pelvic side wall and showing areas liable to surgical damage

The more particular dangers to the ureter during cancer surgery will be dealt with in Volume 3 of the Atlas, but some general references should be made to Figure 3 which shows the course of the ureter and its relationship to blood vessels.

There are three points of potential danger to the pelvic ureter during hysterectomy or pelvic surgery and these are indicated by the numbers 1, 2 and 3 (Figure 3). At 1 the ureter lies in the base of the infundibulopelvic ligament and unless care is exercised in clamping that structure, the ureter can be caught up and damaged or divided. Therefore, it is essential to check that the ureter is below and clear of the chosen point of clamping. At point 2 the ureter is extraperitoneal but otherwise uncovered. It is vulnerable and any inflamed, ectopic or malignant structure is liable to adhere to it, displace it and even invade it. In dealing with chronic pelvic inflammation or where there are widespread pelvic adhesions for any reason, this part of the ureter must be in danger. At point 3 the ureter skirts the uterus on each side at a distance of only 2 cm from the cervix and is surrounded by parametrial tissue which represents the inner aspect of the cardinal ligament. The ureter is not visible in this part of its course, it is tethered in position and there is little space between it and the uterus. Minor faults in hysterectomy technique, perhaps compounded by an abnormality of ureteric course or development, can easily result in damage. The particular dangers associated with certain types of hysterectomy are dealt with in the text.

Venous drainage from pelvis

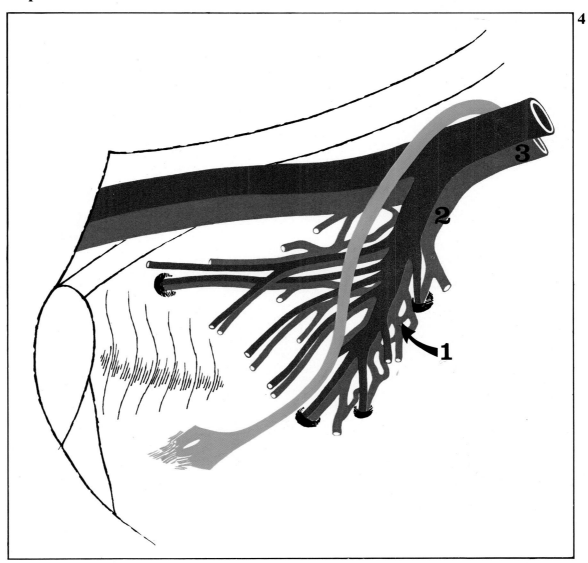

4 Venous drainage from pelvis and its relationship to the ureter

Deep pelvic bleeding is more likely to be a problem in the surgery of malignancy but since it is never possible to know the extent of any operation in advance, the surgeon should be aware of the anatomy of the pelvic blood circulation. This immediately explains why such dangers may arise and shows how they may be avoided.

Figure 4 emphasises the rich venous plexus (1) that drains into the internal (2) and common (3) iliac veins. Not only are the veins much larger and more numerous than the arteries they accompany, but they are also thin-walled with minimal support from the areolar tissue so that they are easily torn. To make matters worse many emerge from the gluteal region and if torn across, the distal ends retract into the pelvic foramina where they cannot be secured by forceps or stitches and it is not even possible to obtain haemostasis by pressure. In this context the surgeon may feel that in the ultimate he always has recourse to ligation of the internal iliac artery on the affected side or on both sides (see page 258). Unhappily, even that may avail him little. The bleeding from this area is largely venous and as there is a very rich collateral circulation through the sacro-sciatic foramen bleeding may persist.

The moral is clear. One must not get involved with the hypogastric venous plexus posterior or deep to the line of the ureter. Only in relatively advanced malignancy should it be necessary to approach this region; that particular problem will be considered in Volume 3.

Surgical instruments

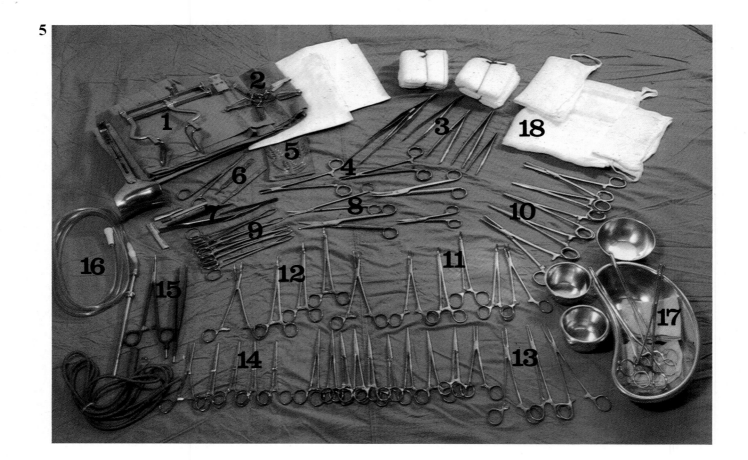

5

The authors' views on surgical equipment were discussed in the Introduction to the Atlas. The general abdominal set in use at the Jessop Hospital for Women, Sheffield, is shown in Figure 5, but most readers will be accustomed to their own choice of instruments and there is no desire to dissuade them from that choice. Those illustrated are of the simplest possible design and have been developed for standard hospital use over a number of years by a succession of exceedingly good and careful surgeons.

For identification purposes we have attached to some instruments the names we have learnt to associate with them, but we fully expect that some readers will recognise these items as those they have always linked with the name of someone else. Surgeons worldwide are aware of these discrepancies. We do not believe that they will be unduly perturbed by seeing their old favourites sailing under an alien flag.

Difficulties encountered in ordering hospital replacements are generally resolved by the instrument makers. They have great pride in their craft and invariably know the origins and development of each instrument.

Figure 5

1 Self-retaining retractor
2 Towel clips
3 Dissecting forceps
4 Needle holders
5 Assorted needles
6 Scalpels
7 Michel clip forceps
8 Scissors
9 Littlewood's forceps
10 Straight Oschner forceps
11 Curved Oschner forceps
12 Miles-Phillips' forceps
13 Allis' tissue forceps
14 Spencer-Wells forceps
15 Diathermy forceps
16 Sucker
17 Sponge forceps and catheterisation equipment
18 Intra-abdominal packs and swabs

2: Opening and closing the abdomen

The choice of abdominal incision for gynaecological work is obviously of great importance. While the prime consideration is to gain adequate access to the operative field, trauma to the abdominal wall should be avoided and postoperative wound complications should be minimal. The resultant scar should be strong and durable.

Until comparatively recently the standard gynaecological approach, in the United Kingdom at least, was a lower midline incision from just below the umbilicus to the symphysis pubis. If wider access were required, it was extended upwards by curving round or cutting through the umbilicus. Some preferred a paramedian incision which could bypass the umbilicus when necessary and at the same time give a marginally stronger scar.

There are several serious objections to these vertical incisions. They are uncomfortable postoperatively and are liable to dehiscence in the presence of infection, distention or malnutrition. Incisional herniae develop much too frequently, especially in obese patients. This is explained by the inherent weakness of the very narrow linea alba and absence of a posterior rectus sheath at this particular level. Even when clinically sound many of these scars are both wide and aesthetically displeasing. The increased incidence of postoperative pulmonary and thromboembolic complications associated with vertical as opposed to transverse incisions is a strong argument against the use of the former.

Gynaecologists have been aware of the transverse alternative but have rather reserved it for its cosmetic advantage when no great degree of access was required. It can take considerably longer to open the abdomen transversely if one is not accustomed to it and unless the wound is closed meticulously, haematomata do occur. Therefore, it is not surprising that it has taken some time for the transverse incision to become established as the standard gynaecological approach, although we believe it has now become so. The transverse incision is incomparably the better incision of the two; with experience it need not be tedious to the surgeon nor give him inferior access in any situation.

The main advantages of the transverse incision at the various levels are as follows.

1 Skin

The incision lies in the natural crease or cleavage line of the skin so that when the incision has been made, the wound edges lie together without tension. When sutured there is no tension whatsoever and this consistently gives a narrow firm scar.

2 Fascia

At fascial level the dense anterior sheath of the rectus is stitched together transversely and is immensely strong. Even in the midline at the linea alba there is dense fibrous tissue. There is little or no muscle pull on the edges and as the recti muscles contract they have the effect of approximating the fascial edges rather than separating them. There is thus no reason for the stitches to cut out or tear out under tension.

3 Muscle

There is no division of actual muscle tissue so that the closure is not only strong but the recti muscles are preserved intact. They remain side by side and are not disturbed in their maintenance of abdominal wall support. They are not in any way impeded in standing up to the most vigorous coughing, retching and unguarded movement in the postoperative phase.

4 Blood supply

The blood supply to the abdominal wall is on a segmental basis with an excellent collateral and anastomotic circulation as far forwards as the midline anteriorly. Only in the vertical plane anteriorly is the blood supply in any way deficient. In the lower abdomen the superficial and deep epigastric vessels anastomose with the superficial and deep circumflex iliac branches to maintain a rich blood supply which encourages wound healing.

5 Nerve supply

The nerve supply of the abdominal wall is also on a segmental basis. Apart from the fact that there is no danger of denervation there is minimal incision of nerve fibres, because the tissues are cut in the line of the nerve distribution. Postoperative comfort is greatly affected and the absence of pain makes early movement and ambulation possible. The secure and uninhibited abdominal wall allows free breathing and clearing of the air passages, thus greatly diminishing the incidence of chest complications.

The only valid criticism of the incision is the tendency to postoperative haematoma formation and occasional haemorrhage. Such complications are almost always the result of errors in technique; if the method described in the text is followed the incidence should be minimal. Since employing the transverse incision to the exclusion of others, we have not seen one case of burst abdomen on a very busy surgical unit.

Lower abdominal transverse incision

The normal or usual transverse incision such as would be used in an abdominal hysterectomy operation will be described in detail. Variations to suit individual situations in gynaecological practice will then be referred to.

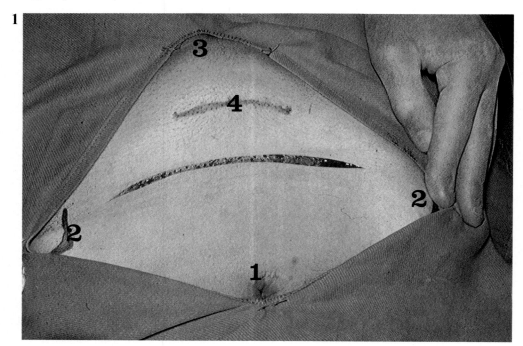

Transverse incision: opening the abdomen

1 Skin incision

In the illustration the incision has been made in the skin crease approximately 4 cm above the pubic crest, slightly concave upwards and about 12 cm in length. The ends are approximately 3 cm below the anterior superior iliac spines. Skin markings and numbers are used as reference viz: umbilicus (1), anterior superior iliac spines (2), and symphysis pubis (3). The skin marking (4) indicates the placing of the short low incision for lesser pelvic surgery (page 27).

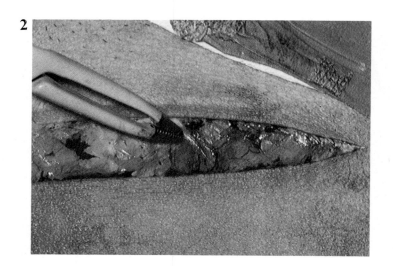

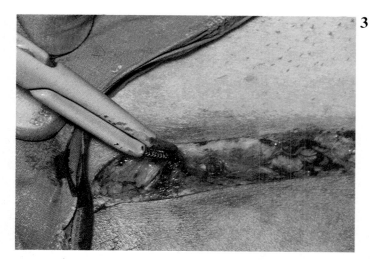

2 and 3 Superficial haemostasis

Some bleeding is inevitable as the skin incision is made but unless the superficial epigastric vessels are divided, this can be disregarded in the first place as the vessels are otherwise cutaneous. To touch them with the diathermy will lead to charring of the skin edge with unsightly crusts and scarring during healing. The superficial epigastric vessels are towards the lateral aspect of the wound and only about 7 cm apart, so that they have to be dealt with to give adequate access. If already cut the ends are picked up carefully and sealed with diathermy; otherwise these vessels are exposed from the fat with the diathermy forceps and sealed before dividing them. They can of course be clamped, cut and tied. In Figure 2 the right superficial epigastric artery is being sealed; in Figure 3 the left artery is being sealed.

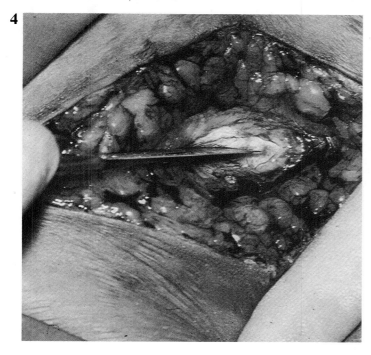

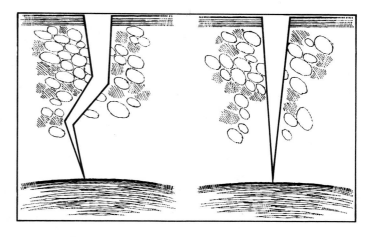

Incorrect   **Correct**

4 Incision of superficial and deep fascia

The full depth of the fat is incised down to the rectus sheath but only in about the central 3 or 4 cm of the skin wound. This is done with one stroke of the scalpel with the left hand steadying the wound area so that there is no sideways slip; this results in a clean wound face. A series of cuts causes an irregular staircase effect which makes accurate approximation impossible and encourages haematomata. Compare the diagrams above where the advantages of 2 over 1 are obvious.

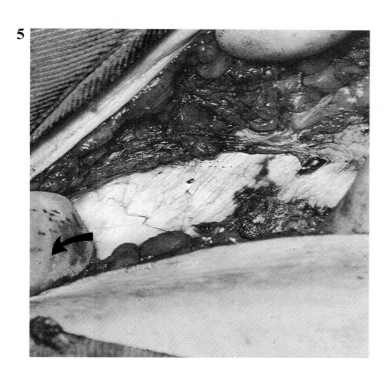

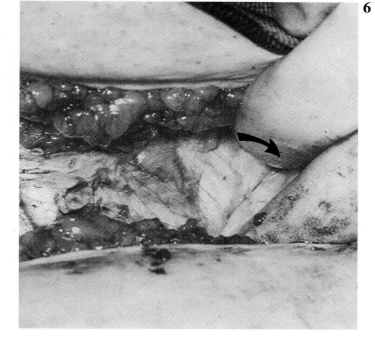

5 and 6 Enlargement of incision by lateral digital retraction

With the forefinger close to the rectus sheath aponeurosis first on one side and then the other, superficial and deep fascial layers are separated in the line of the wound by pulling laterally in the direction of the arrows to widen it to the full extent. This allows wide access to the rectus sheath without bleeding from the small arteries which are either pulled laterally out of the way and left intact, or if they are torn their retracting intima seals them.

7

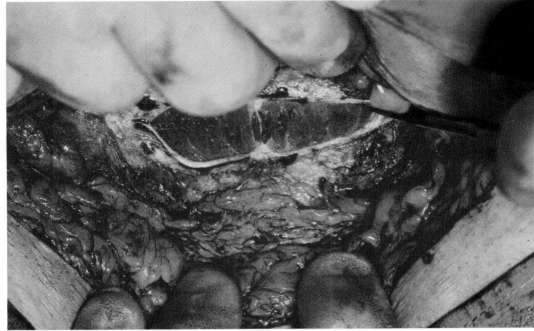

7 Incision of anterior rectus sheath
With a gentle stroke of the scalpel the rectus sheath is opened transversely in the median part on each side of the midline and this displays the vertical fibres of the recti and the central linea alba.

8

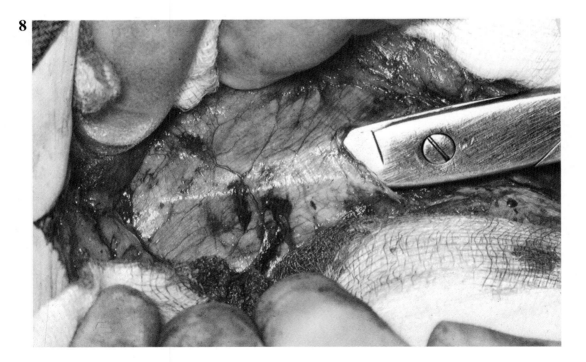

8 Lateral extension of rectus sheath incision
The incision in the rectus sheath is carried transversely as far as the lateral edge of each rectus muscle. Curved scissors are used. It is essential first to insert the scissors with closed blades between the rectus sheath and the muscle to ensure separation before cutting. Unless this definition of the sheath is made the superficial fibres of the muscle will inevitably be cut transversely thus weakening the muscle and giving a very untidy effect.

9

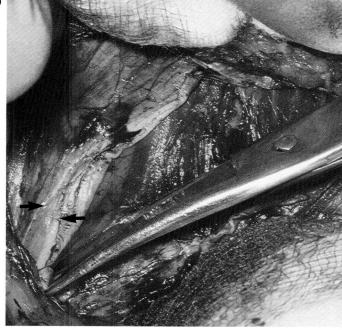

10

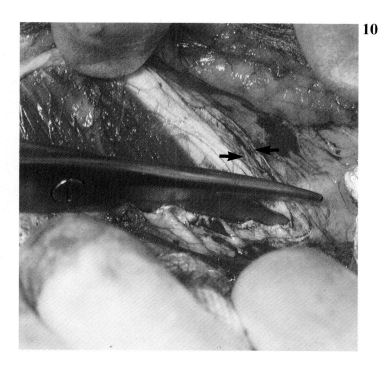

9 and 10 Transverse opening of rectus sheath

When the lateral edge of the rectus muscle has been seen the incision should not be extended further, otherwise bleeding will be encountered. In Figure 9 the left rectus sheath is fully incised and the two layers of fascia in the lateral half of the sheath are indicated by arrows. In Figure 10 the same stage has been reached on the right and again the external and internal oblique layers are arrowed.

11

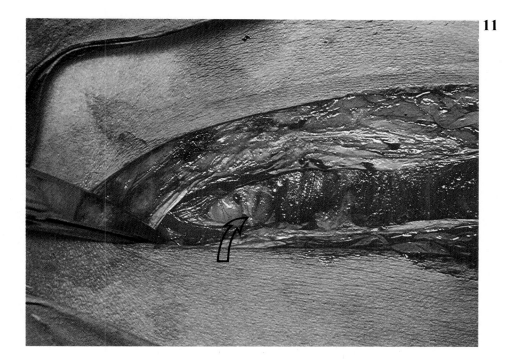

11 Deep epigastric vessels

This photograph is cautionary and shows fairly large branches of the deep epigastric vessels (arrowed) which will give troublesome bleeding if the wound is opened too far laterally.

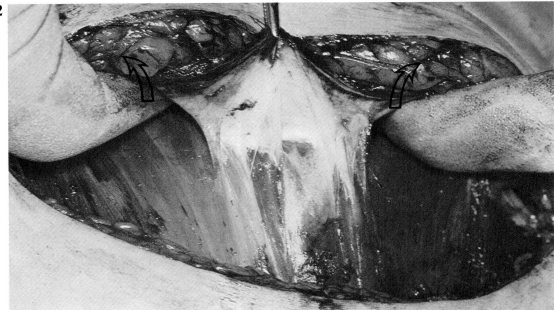

12 Freeing anterior rectus sheath from underlying muscles (1)

The edge of the upper leaf of the anterior rectus sheath is held in Spencer Wells forceps at its midpoint and raised off the linea alba and recti muscles. With the finger the muscle is carefully separated off the sheath lateral to the midline in the direction of the arrows. Care is taken not to cause bleeding by tearing the perforating branches of the deep epigastric arteries. The inner edges of the recti remain adherent to the linea alba and to the sheath so that it is necessary to separate the sheath by sharp dissection before proceeding further.

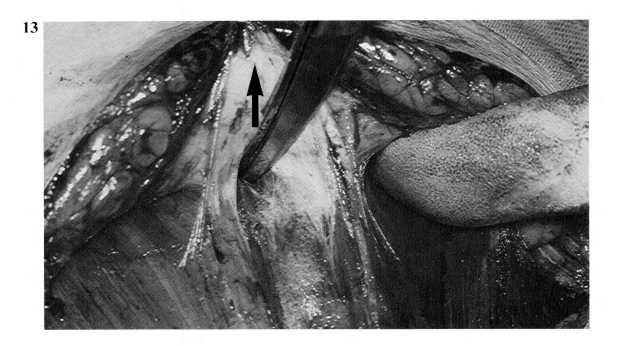

13 Freeing anterior rectus sheath from underlying muscles (2)

The sheath is released in an upwards direction with scissor cuts as shown (arrowed) and the recti muscles fall back from the raised sheath.

14

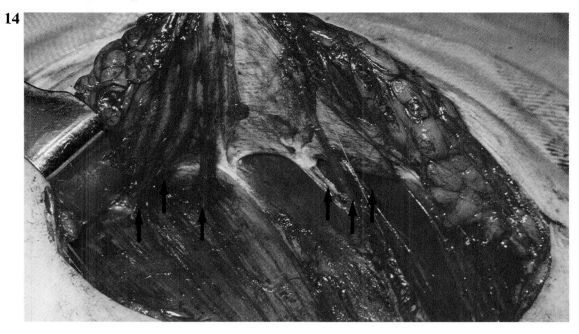

14 Securing perforating branches of deep epigastric artery

The perforating branches of the deep epigastric vessels are shown entering the under surface of the rectus sheath and this appearance is very constant. The illustration shows exactly where they can be expected to lie and it is not proposed to attempt to describe them, but to indicate the usual six points with arrows. They can be sealed off with diathermy conveniently and easily.

15

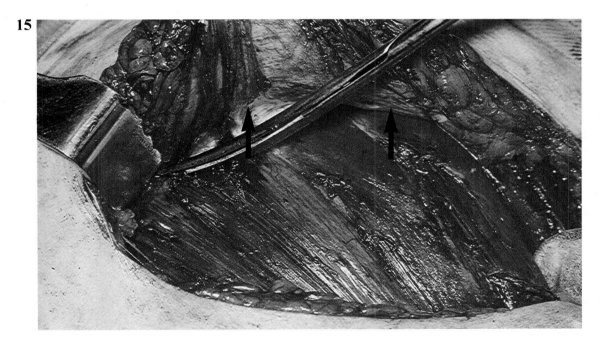

15 Dividing the vascular and other attachments to the rectus sheath

The vessels are shown being divided with scissors and fine fibrous attachments are also cut so that the sheath can be elevated off the recti muscles. Continuing separation upwards in the direction of the arrows allows it to be raised as far as the umbilicus without hindrance. This means that the incision can occupy the whole distance between the symphysis pubis and the umbilicus, resulting in an available length of no less than in a vertical incision.

16
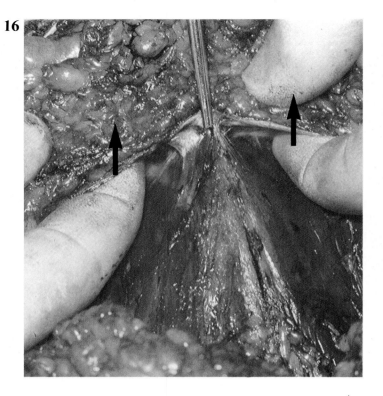

17
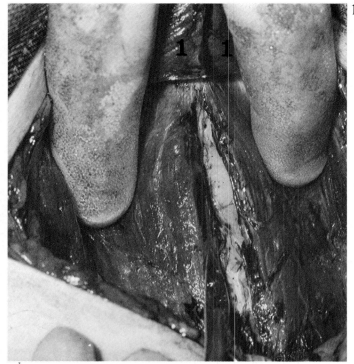

16 and 17 Freeing the anterior rectus sheath (lower leaf)

The centre of the lower leaf is held with Spencer Wells forceps and the fingers are used to separate it from the anterior aspect of the muscles as arrowed in Figure 16. The central attachment of the sheath to the recti muscles is firm and must be divided by scissors to enter a plane of cleavage which is sometimes superficial and sometimes deep to the pyramidalis muscle. In this instance it is deep to the muscles (1 and 1).

18
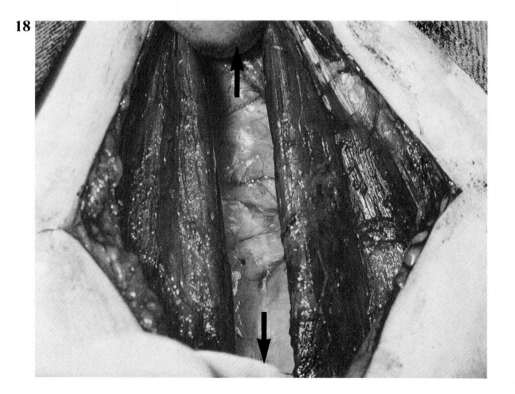

18 Separation of recti muscles

The assistant holds the leaves of the rectus sheath apart to display the muscles in the whole of the sub-umbilical length. These are separated in the midline with the scalpel. Since the peritoneum is loose and falls away from the scalpel there is no danger of entering the peritoneal cavity. The fingers are then inserted between the bellies of the muscles which are separated by pulling longitudinally as arrowed. Slight lateral displacement of the muscles then gives adequate exposure of the underlying peritoneum before incision.

19

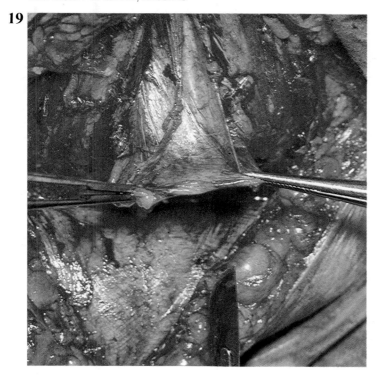

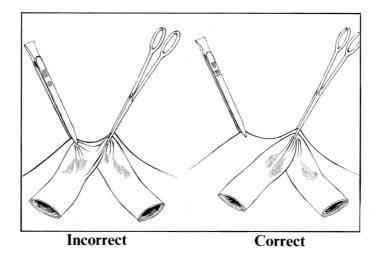

Incorrect   **Correct**

19 to 21 Opening the peritoneal cavity

The loose peritoneum at the middle of the wound is picked up by forceps at least 1 cm lateral to the midline on each side and held ready for incision by scalpel or scissors as shown in Figure 19. It is important that the forceps be well apart. If they are too close together and each is immobilising the same loop of bowel, it will be cut into as the peritoneum is held taut for incision. The diagrams (1 and 2) show the danger and how it can be avoided. In Figure 20 a further safety measure is used. The taut fold is palpated between forefinger and thumb before incision to exclude the presence of underlying structures. Figure 21 shows the scalpel opening the peritoneal cavity.

20

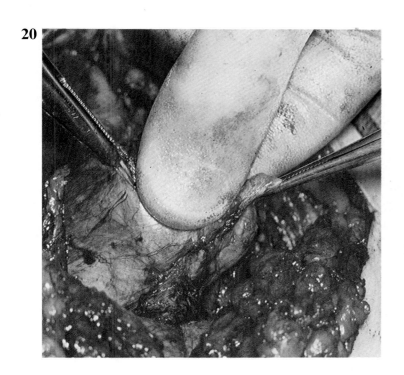

21

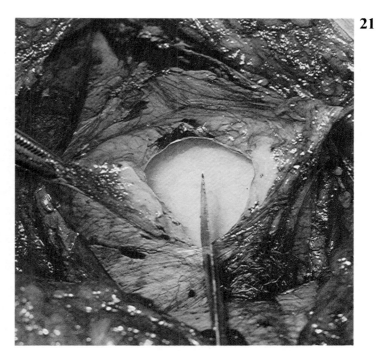

22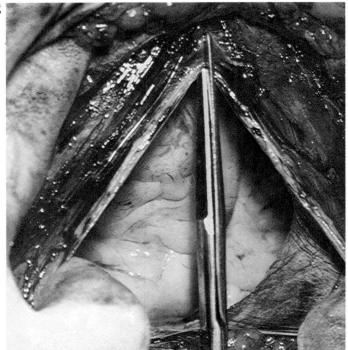

23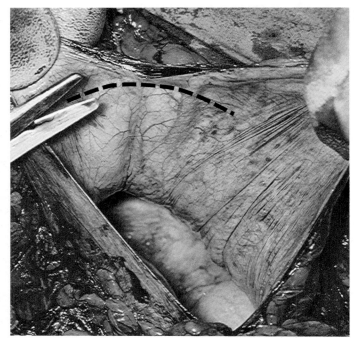

24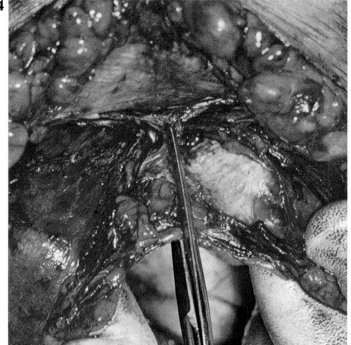

22 to 24 Enlarging the peritoneal opening

Surgeon and assistant each insert a forefinger into the peritoneal cavity to support the peritoneum well clear of the viscera. The incision is extended towards the lower end of the wound with the scissors as shown in Figure 22. The opening is limited by the presence of the bladder and the under surface of the peritoneum is carefully examined by the surgeon to distinguish the upper edge of the bladder. Light is not transmitted through the two relatively thick layers of the bladder wall whereas the peritoneum is easily trans-illuminated above it; this clearly indicates the limit of the incision. In Figure 23 the upper border of the bladder is outlined by a broken line. As this incision is made, minor bleeding may be encountered on the peritoneal edge and it is better dealt with immediately. Surgeon and assistant then reverse the direction of their fingers to support the peritoneum in the upper half of the wound and that is opened by scissors as shown in Figure 24. There should be no bleeding at this stage of the operation.

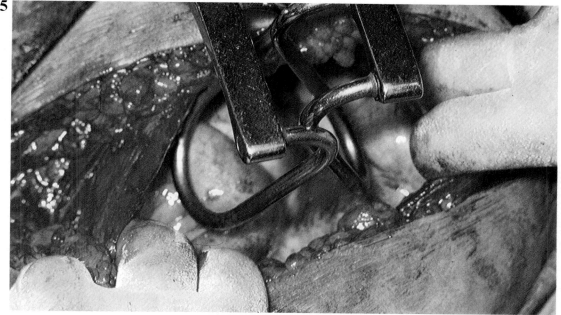

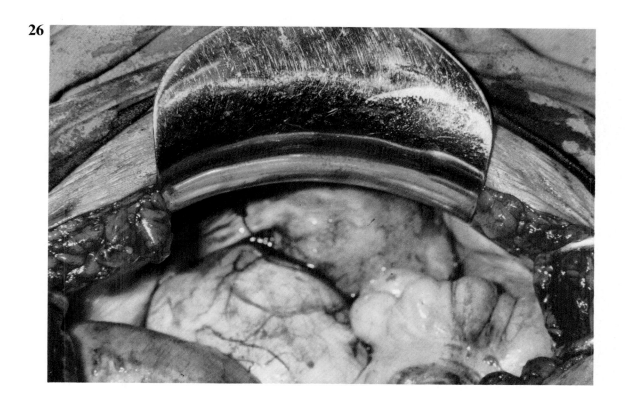

25 and 26 Preliminary examination and placing of self-retaining retractor

The use of a Balfour's self-retaining retractor is shown and described as standard procedure in the Atlas. Some gynaecologists prefer a large Doyen's retractor; others favour a four-bladed retractor. All are satisfactory and are a matter of personal preference. It is at this stage of the operation that the surgeon will wish to insert his hand into the peritoneal cavity to make a general examination of the viscera. Such an examination is not facilitated by the presence of firm metal retractors; their placement is better postponed until the examination has been made.

27

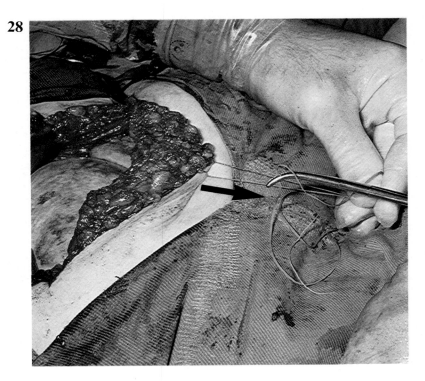

27 Packing off the intestine and omentum during operation

It is usual to tilt the operating table into a Trendelenburg or head down position at this stage; the degree of tilt is a matter for the surgeon. A steep tilt greatly aids access by enabling the bowel and omentum to retreat into the upper abdomen, but the anaesthetist may well object if the patient is on assisted respiration or under epidural analgesia. In such instances a compromise must be found. Most surgeons use a large moist abdominal pack to keep the abdominal contents from the field of operation as shown here. In the oblique view in the illustration (27) the uterus (1) is being held up and forwards while a retractor (2) lifts the upper wound edge to show the pack (3) restraining the abdominal contents.

28

28 Improving access in the obese patient

Many patients have a thick abdominal wall and a redundant roll of fat in the upper leaf of the wound edge which obtrudes on the surgeon's view. This is best dealt with as shown in the illustration. A stitch is taken through the apex of the skin flap at two points to avoid cutting through the tissues. The suture is long so that the two ends can be thrown clear in a cephalad direction, as arrowed, and fixed to the operating table. This keeps the flap clear of the wound and allows better access.

Lower abdominal transverse incision: variations in differing circumstances

The technique of the operation varies only in the size and placing of the incision. In minor operations where no great degree of access is necessary the incision can be quite short and within the pubic hairline at approximately 2 cm from the pubic crest as indicated by the skin marking on Figure 1 (page **16**). Where there is a very large abdominal mass to be removed or good access is essential, as in a Wertheim hysterectomy, the incision is set higher so that it can be carried as far laterally as required and so that access to the region of the pelvic brim is satisfactory.

29

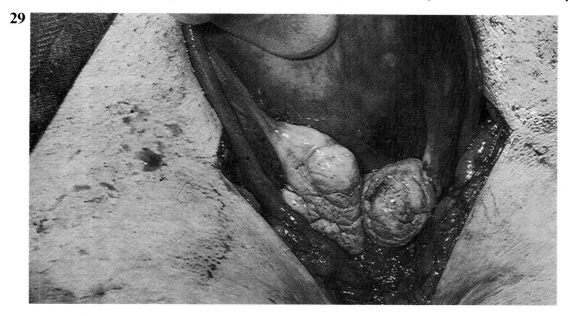

30

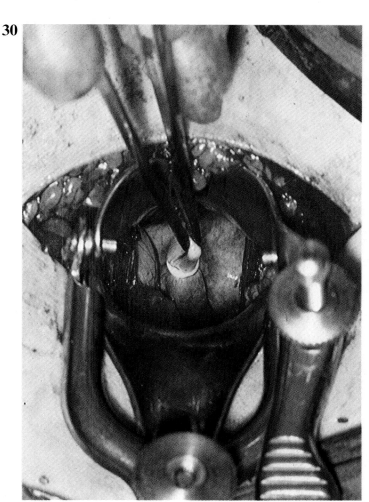

29 Short suprapubic incision for lesser gynaecological operations

The level of the incision in this instance is 2 cm above the symphysis pubis and the length is 5 cm. The uterus is held up between fingers and thumb and the upper edge of the wound is retracted in a cephalad direction to give clear access to tubes and ovaries. Access is more than adequate for tubal ligation and allows for any lesser pelvic operation being done.

30 'Minilap' type incision

The incision is placed at the same level but is even shorter and could indeed be shorter and still accommodate the 'minilap' retractor or be held open by fine retractors. This kind of incision allows for placing Falope rings (as illustrated), or clips, or for diathermy sterilisation.

31

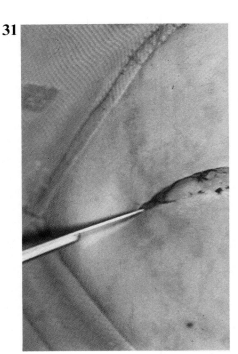

32

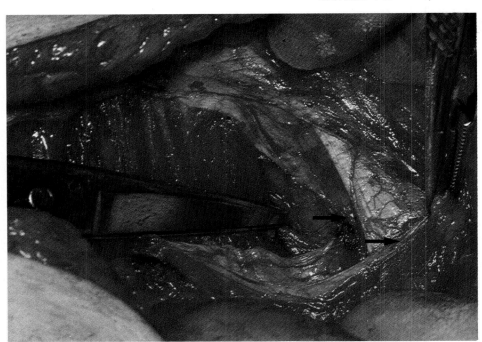

31 to 33 High wide transverse incision

The group of cases referred to on page **27** includes patients with large ovarian cysts which may be malignant and therefore have to be removed intact. It is important to ensure adequate exposure. The skin incision is approximately 6 cm from the pubic crest and curves out naturally in the skin crease to clear the anterior superior iliac spines. It can therefore be taken as far towards the loin as required. The apex of the drapes in Figure 31 lies over the left anterior superior iliac spine and indicates the line of the incision. In Figure 32 the lateral edge of the right rectus muscle is defined; the arrows indicate where the fascial and muscular

33

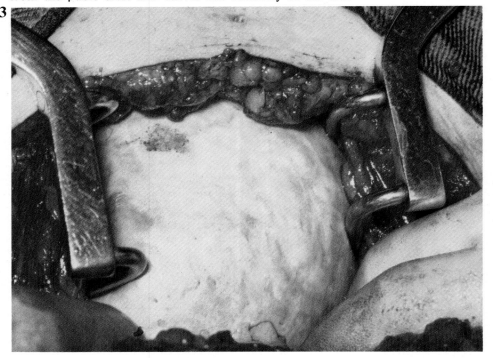

components of the abdominal wall are incised if further access is required. The charred area indicates where branches of the inferior epigastric or deep circumflex iliac artery have been encountered and sealed off with diathermy. Figure 33 indicates the wide access becoming available as a self-retaining retractor is inserted.

Transverse incision: closing the abdomen

When the operation has been completed and haemostasis checked, the large abdominal pack is retrieved and the self-retaining retractor removed. The theatre or 'scrub' nurse now commences her check of the swab and instrument count and will report to the surgeon before the peritoneum is closed. In the meantime the surgeon ensures that the viscera assume their normal position and draws down the omentum as a protective apron over the operation field. The edges of the peritoneum are picked up by forceps and the wound is ready for closure.

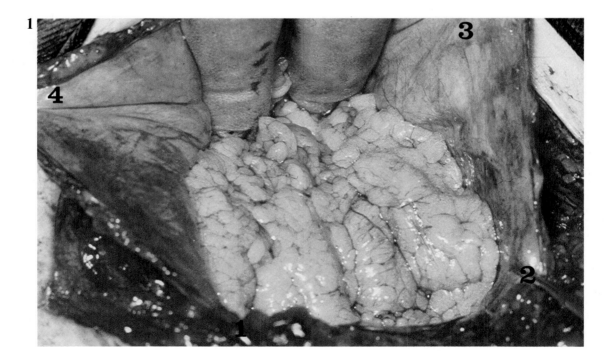

1 Wound ready for closure

The abdomen is about to be closed and the lower edge of the wound is retracted by the fingers to show that there is adequate free peritoneum. Four points, (1), (2), (3) and (4), are picked up with Spencer-Wells forceps to delineate the edges clearly.

2

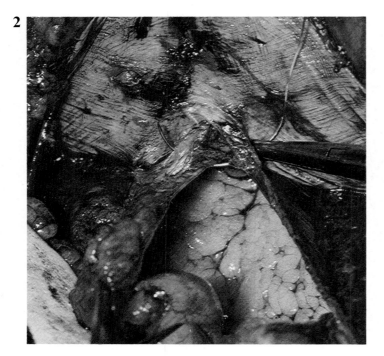

3

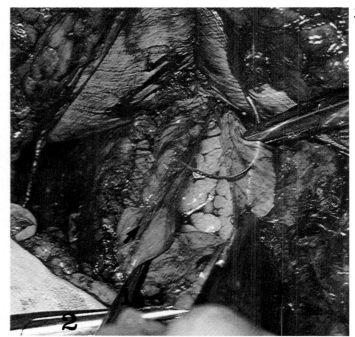

2 Peritoneal closure (1)

A round-bodied needle carrying a PGA No. 0 suture commences closure of the peritoneal opening just below the umbilicus. It is possible to obtain a firm fibrous edge of peritoneum on each side because it is above the level of the semi-circular line and thus there is a posterior rectus sheath. Transversalis fascia is adherent to the peritoneum and was incised with it when the upper part of the wound was opened. The needle is seen to pick up a good bite of tissue on each side giving a strong anchor and commencement to the continuous stitch.

3 Peritoneal closure (2)

The continuous suture is now below the level of the semi-circular line and the thin and unsupported peritoneum is seen. Sometimes it is easily buttonholed or torn by the needle and in such cases closure can be strengthened by taking a loop or double transfixion on each side as the stitch proceeds; this procedure is shown. There is also a thin layer representing transversalis fascia just lateral and under the edge of the recti muscles and it can be included to strengthen the peritoneal stitch. The layers are arrowed; that on the right is easily visible and the left is seen just lateral to the dissecting forceps (3). The numerals 1 and 2 indicate the forceps on the lower half of the peritoneal opening which have been crossed over each other to bring the edges together.

4

5

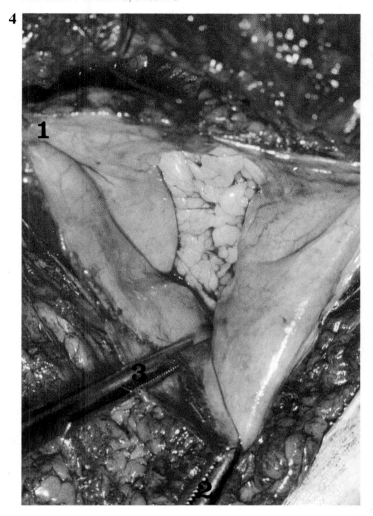

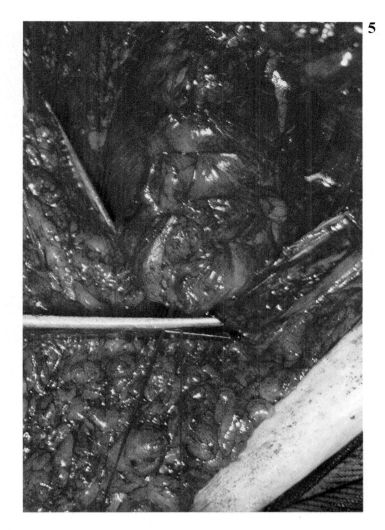

4 and 5 Peritoneal closure (3)

The lateral retaining forceps 1 and 2 are being replaced by a single forceps (3) on the very lowest edge of the peritoneal opening so that it can be lifted up to ensure complete closure as shown in Figure 4. In Figure 5 the peritoneum is finally closed with the suture tied beyond the holding forceps and the stitch is shown being cut short. The closed peritoneum falls back below the level of the recti muscles and the suture line is examined for haemostasis and security.

6

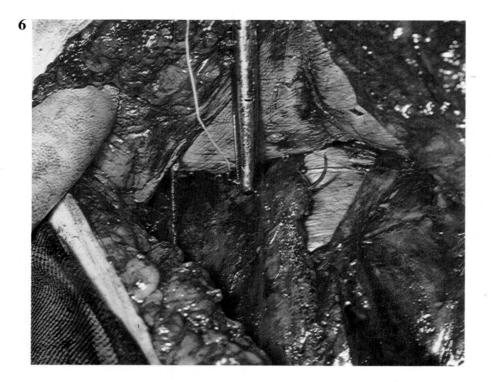

6 and 7 Approximation of recti muscles

There is some doubt whether it is necessary to bring together the medial edges of the recti muscles, but it is noticeable as in Figure 6 that they do not always assume a satisfactory side-to-side position if left to themselves. We think it is correct to approximate them by two fine PGA No. 00 sutures tied loosely so as to approximate the medial edges, yet in no sense to compress or cut into the muscle tissue. This has been done in Figure 7.

7

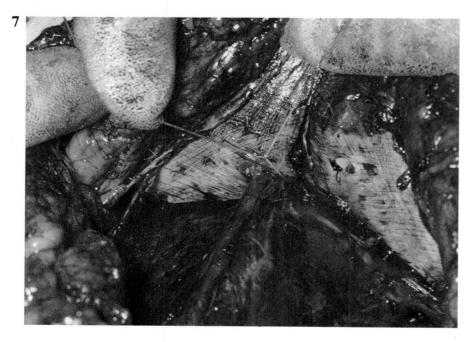

8

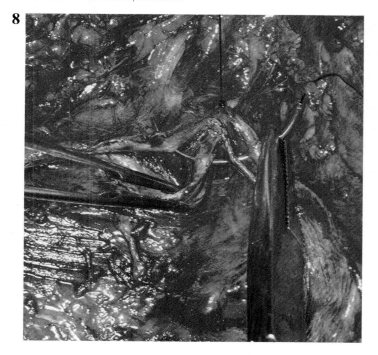

9

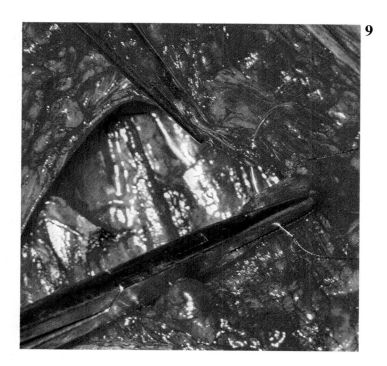

8, 9 and 10 Closure of anterior rectus sheath

With the skin flaps gently retracted by Littlewood's forceps the rectus sheath is closed by a transverse overlapping continuous PGA No. 1 suture carried on an atraumatic needle. In Figure 8 the anchor suture has been tied and the short end cut off. The needle has already picked up the two

layers of the upper edge of the sheath in the right angle of the wound and is transfixing the two layers of the lower edge. Note how the deeper layer of the lower sheath retracts behind the anterior layer and has to be actively sought. It is very easy to omit a layer at this stage and that only results in a weak scar. In Figure 9 the closure has proceeded to a point where the two

10

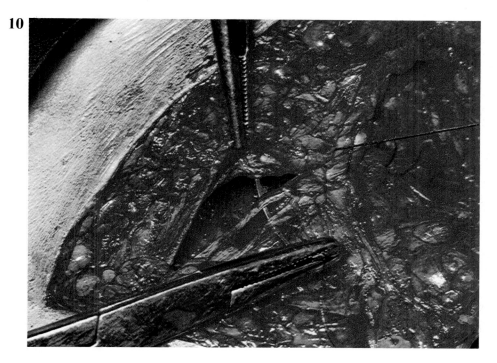

layers have become fused and this continues across the midline. On the opposite side in Figure 10 the two layers are again definitively picked up from both upper and lower sheaths; the stitch continues laterally until the wound is completely closed. The final stitch pierces the external oblique only, is tied off and is cut short.

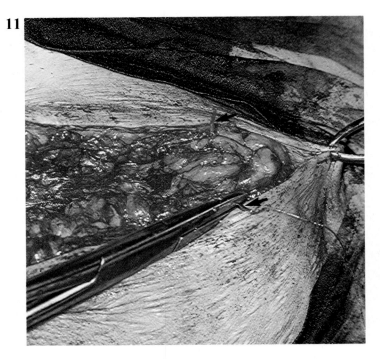

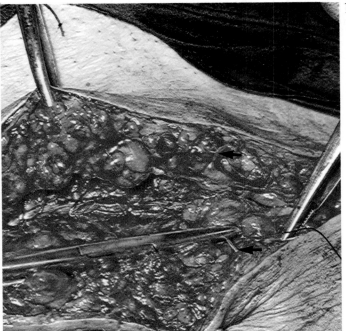

11 to 13 Closure of deep fascia

To avoid haematomata from small vessels it is essential with these incisions to eliminate all dead space in the wound. The importance of a smooth wound 'face' has been emphasised, but it is also necessary in an area of loose tissue planes to leave no space into which blood may collect. The stitch used to

effect this is a fine PGA No. 00 suture on a round-bodied needle; its purpose is to approximate the cut deep fascia although it takes in some of the deeper superficial fascial layer also. The stitch must be carefully placed and should not be too tight lest it distort the wound or cause compression of fat. The wound should be properly splinted before the stitch is placed;

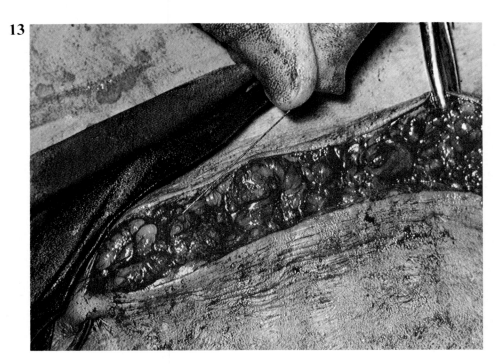

this is done by applying a Littlewood's forceps lateral to each angle of the skin wound and keeping these taut by lateral pull during closure. In Figure 11 the needle has picked up the upper layer of deep fascia and is ready to penetrate the lower edge. Note that a certain amount of fatty tissue is taken so that approximation is cushioned from being too tight. The suture

continues across the wound as shown in Figure 12 and in Figure 13 the stitch has been tied off.

Skin closure

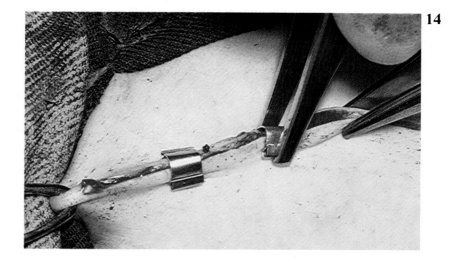

14

It is not proposed to go into the question of preferred methods of closing the skin. There are many satisfactory ways of doing so, and we favour Michel's clips which can be removed on the fifth day and leave no permanent mark. If there is any question of tension on the wound, if the patient is very obese or if there is the possibility of infection then PGA No. 00 suture in the form of interrupted stitches is more suitable. These do not need to be removed and they are easily rubbed off when the buried part of the sutures has been absorbed. If frank sepsis has been encountered during operation and especially if drains have been inserted it is wise to use monofilmament unabsorbable suture, usually placed as interrupted vertical mattress stitches. Some prefer to use a continuous subcuticular stitch especially with the lesser gynaecological operations, but the method is more suitable

for use in the upper abdomen where the skin is supported by denser subcutaneous tissue with a firm wound edge. In the lower abdomen the tissues are lax with loose superficial fascia and there is a tendency for the skin to be redundant. If used in the lower abdomen this type of suture is better restricted to very young women with firm tissues.

14 Skin closure with Michel's clips
Double clips are being applied and should be at a distance of 2 cm from each other to avoid sealing the wound and allow the escape of any blood which may have oozed from the edges. The clips are removed by forceps designed for the purpose on the fourth or fifth postoperative day.

15

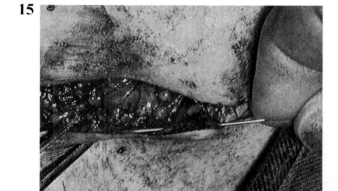

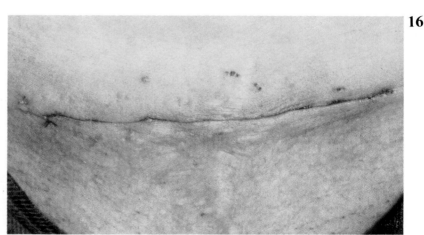

16

15 and 16 Subcuticular skin closure
The method of picking up the skin edge with a straight needle carrying a PGA No. 00 suture is shown. The wound edges are held taut with forceps to give accurate closure and to give a symmetrical effect. The needle is subcutaneous rather than subcuticular (Figure 15). The closed wound is seen in Figure 16.

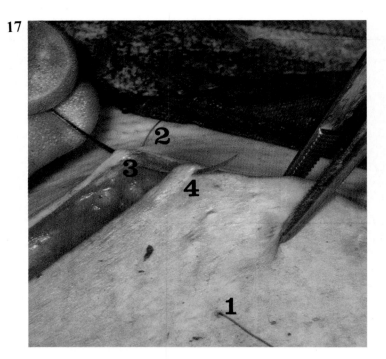

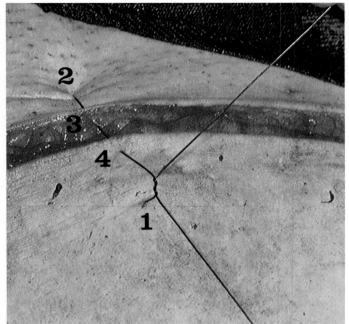

17 and 18 Skin closure in infected cases

These illustrations show the method of using monofilament suture as a vertical mattress stitch. In Figure 17 the progression of the needle is numbered (1) to (4) and the principle is to obtain deep closure while at the same time bringing the skin edges into neat apposition. The stitch is being tied in Figure 18 and the double first hitch will be observed.

Lower abdominal midline vertical incision

The authors recognise that many surgeons and gynaecologists still prefer the vertical incision. They have been trained in its use, it has given very satisfactory results and although not perfect they are not prepared to abandon it for an incision which also has its own shortcomings. The incision illustrated is a lower midline vertical one which in most respects serves as a model for paramedian also. The steps which the incisions have in common will be illustrated but not described. In following the description and illustrations the reader will have to take into account whether he himself usually operates from the right or left side of the patient. The operation is shown as being done from the left side but the upper and lower ends of the wound are identified with markers where there is any ambiguity.

Opening the abdomen (vertical incision)

1 Skin incision
Steadying the skin of the lower abdomen with the forefinger and thumb of the left hand a midline straight incision is made from the mons pubis just above the symphysis to just below the umbilicus. The incision is through skin but inevitably includes a certain amount of superficial fascia. Note the two transverse scratches on the skin made with the back of the scalpel before incision and as a guide to neat apposition when closing the wound. There is no great amount of bleeding at this stage and no attempt is made at haemostasis.

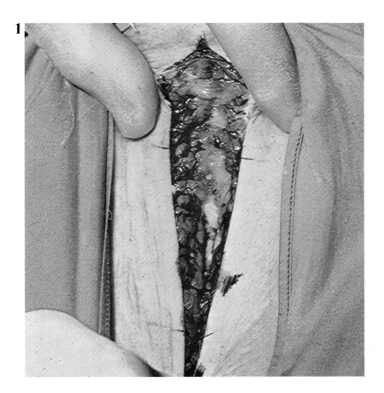

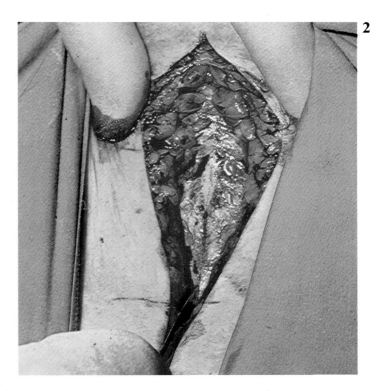

2 Incision through superficial and deep fascia
Continuing to steady the wound in the same way the incision is taken through the superficial and deep fascia to expose the rectus sheath in the length of the wound. As in the transverse incision the aim should be to do this in one stroke and so retain a smooth wound face. There are usually some small bleeding vessels at this stage; these are either sealed with diathermy or tied off with fine suture material.

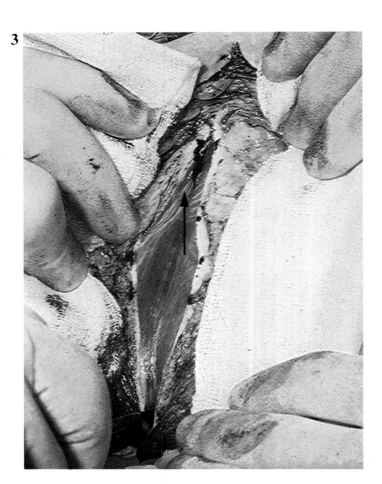

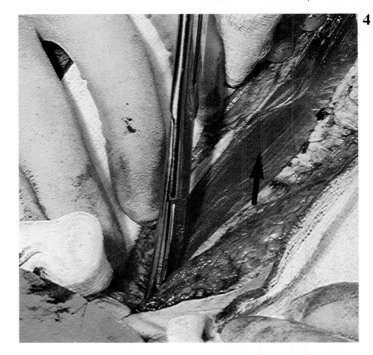

3 Incision of rectus sheath

The incision is continued in the midline through the rectus sheath and will expose one or other rectus muscle in part of the incision at least. In this instance the left rectus muscle has been exposed and the edge of the sheath falls away to expose the left rectus muscle. Any doubts about which side is entered are resolved by seeing the line of the pyramidalis muscle fibres in the lower part of the wound (arrowed).

4 Opening the left rectus sheath

With curved scissors the sheath is opened up in the length of the incision to expose the muscle (arrowed) and the cut edge falls laterally. The medial edge of the muscle comes into view as it falls away from the linea alba indicating that the incision is almost exactly median.

5 Opening the right rectus sheath

The scalpel is used to incise the right rectus sheath and expose the edge of the right rectus muscle. As the scalpel is drawn towards the umbilicus the lateral edge of the right sheath is seen falling outwards. Both recti muscles retract from the midline and the extra peritoneal fat becomes visible between them in the lower part of the wound.

6

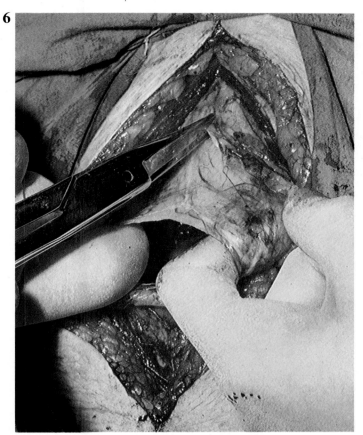

7

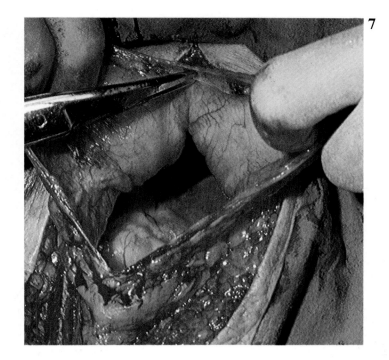

8

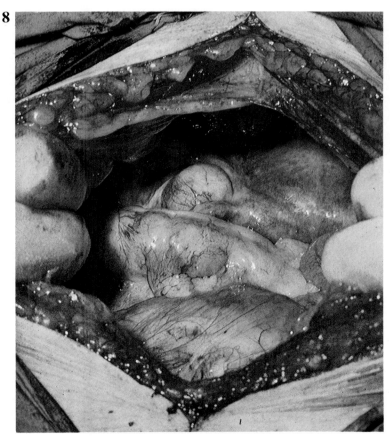

6 to 8 Opening the peritoneal cavity

This procedure is done as in the transverse incision and observing the same precautions in regard to avoidance of potential injury to the bowel. In Figure 6 the extraperitoneal fat is being divided down to the symphysis to expose the peritoneum as far as the bladder. In Figure 7 the peritoneum is incised carefully in a caudad direction as far as the upper border of the bladder and using diathermy to seal the small vessels. In Figure 8 the peritoneum has now been opened in a cephalad direction to just short of the umbilicus. Lateral retraction of the recti muscles brings the pelvic viscera into view.

Weak and deficient lower abdominal scar

The surgeon is frequently confronted by a broad vertical or paramedian scar from a previous pelvic operation. The skin is stretched and thin and there are nearly always weak areas where the recti muscles have pulled laterally and fail to give underlying support. In some instances there is definite ventral herniation. In all such circumstances, and where a further operation is being done, the scar should be excised and the opportunity taken to repair the layers of the abdominal wall.

Repair of the deeper layers is straightforward in that the edges of the peritoneum and the rectus sheath need only be defined laterally to establish strong and smooth edges which are carefully approximated. There is no need to excise tissue. The skin layer is weak, unsightly and poorly vascularised so that it has to be excised. The illustrations show the method and extent of doing so if a narrow and acceptable scar is to be obtained.

9
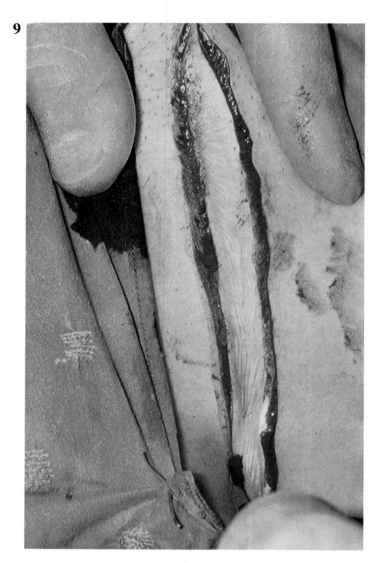

10
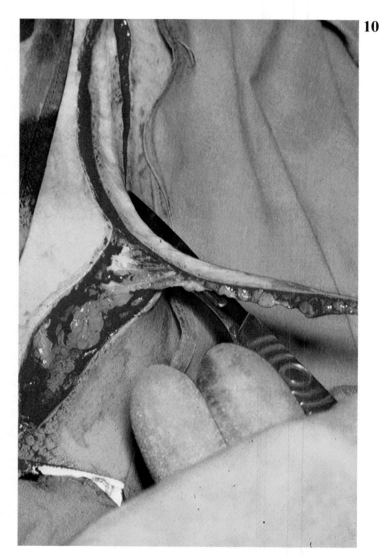

9 Excision of previous scar (1)
In this illustration the scalpel has cut through the skin only, along the right side of the scar and is completing a similar incision on the left side. The line of the incision is 0.5 cm lateral to any area of attenuated skin and is kept on a very slight curve and indeed as nearly straight as possible. The skin of the abdomen is steadied with the thumb and forefinger of the left hand as in previous incisions and the manoeuvre is very much a freehand exercise which should not tax a practical surgeon.

10 Excision of previous scar (2)
The upper end of the skin area is held in a pair of forceps after being detached; the elipse of skin is separated from the underlying tissues throughout its whole length by a series of inward sloping cuts using the scalpel as illustrated, so that a V-shaped and not very deep trench of skin and superficial fascia is taken out over the length of the wound. This subsequently allows accurate skin closure. When this tissue has been removed completely the anterior aspect of the aponeurosis is exposed or covered only by a thin layer of fat.

Closing the abdomen (Vertical incision)

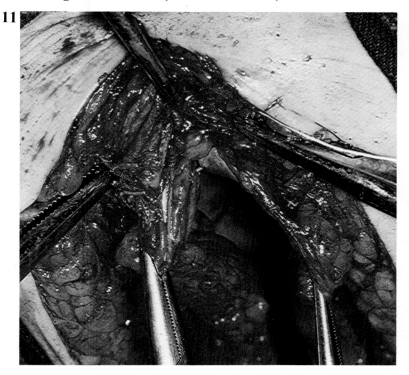
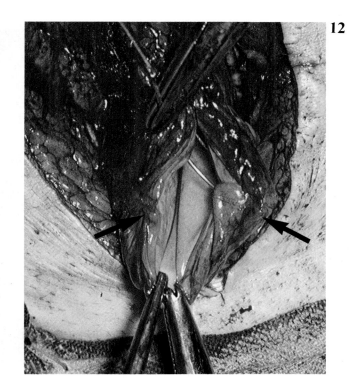

The peritoneum is closed exactly as in the transverse incision and skin suture is essentially the same although there is more strain and pull on a vertical incision and clips may be less satisfactory. If they are used then a deep fascial suture should be used to give support. The rectus sheath is at a disadvantage from straining and must be most carefully approximated with inert and preferably absorbable suture (PGA No. 1 suture on an atraumatic needle is used).

11 and 12 Closure of peritoneum

This procedure is done exactly as in the transverse incision (page 30) but is repeated here because Figure 11 shows the strong peritoneum in the upper part of the wound where it is reinforced by the transversalis fascia above the semicircular line. The thin layer which represents transversalis fascia in the lower part of the wound is clearly seen and is arrowed.

13

14

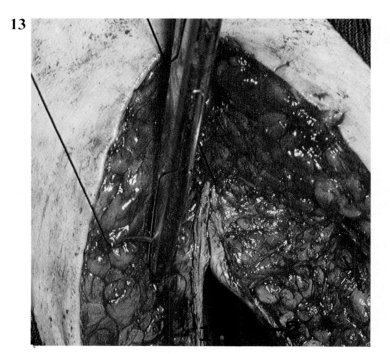

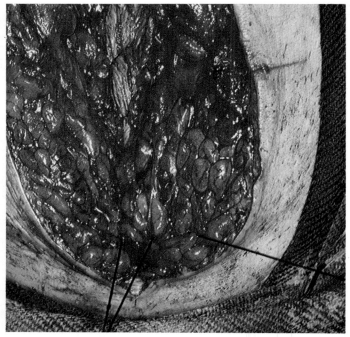

15

13 and 14 Closure of rectus sheath

The edges of the rectus sheath on each side fall together easily and without tension and the edges of the muscles can be seen underneath (1 and 2). A continuous PGA No. 1 suture is used and the stitches are no more than 1.5 cm apart and sufficiently far from the edge as not to be in danger of tearing out. The stitches should not be too tight.

15 Closure of superficial layer

The anchorage of the continuous PGA No. 00 deep fascia suture is being placed and the stitch is continued in the length of the wound without being too tight or the individual stitches too close. The skin is subsequently closed by interrupted vertical mattress stitches of PGA No. 1 suture.

3: Abdominal hysterectomy

Hysterectomy is the most common major operation in gynaecology and the majority of such operations are done abdominally. A proportion are done for malignant disease and these techniques are generally specialised; they are described in Volume 3 of the Atlas. Otherwise the indications for operation include uterine fibroids, endometriosis and chronic inflammatory disease.

In many western countries a sizeable group of indications are listed under the general heading of dysfunctional uterine bleeding. This group is made up of women with anovulatory cycles and irregular heavy bleeding who have not responded to hormone therapy; their inclusion merits some further comment. The number coming to operation for this indication varies greatly in different parts of the world. In Europe hysterectomy is barely acceptable for any such case while in the United States the removal of a troublesome and in the long term possibly dangerous uterus is preferred sooner rather than later. In the United Kingdom an attempt is made to steer a middle course but it must be admitted that decisions are not always completely rational. Courses of hormones vary widely in their adequacy and degree of supervision; many patients are afraid and reluctant to take them for any length of time. Complete menstrual correction and control is expected both currently and in the future. In modern society patients will not have their economic and social lives upset for any length of time. For these reasons demands for hysterectomy are not infrequent and are sometimes difficult to resist. Readers of the Atlas will appreciate that the authors are setting out the various accepted policies as objectively as possible and without any presumption as to whether or not any one is correct.

There is recurring discussion in gynaecological circles throughout the world as to whether or not hysterectomy is done excessively. It must be well nigh impossible to reach any conclusion on such a question. We do not propose to enter into that controversy.

In relation to non-malignant hysterectomy there are always differences of opinion on the question of whether or not to remove or conserve ovaries. There is no easy solution but at the same time reference should be made to points which deserve careful consideration. No woman wants to lose her ovaries unless there is danger in their retention; the fact that she has reached the menopause does not nowadays alter that situation. With so much emotive non-medical discussion on hormone replacement therapy premenopausal and menopausal women tend to develop conservative views about their ovaries. These should generally be respected provided the risks are considered to be very small. It is both tragic and disconcerting when occasionally and usually quite rarely, ovarian carcinoma supervenes, yet reason demands that one should be committed to a sensibly thought out policy. Conservation is generally favoured by the authors but any features suggestive of possible malignant change in an ovary would of course lead to its removal. A rather different view is held in relation to cases of widespread pelvic endometriosis where most surgeons strive to retain at least part of an ovary. The experience of having to reoperate and remove a carefully preserved ovary or part of an ovary because of continuing pain is not infrequent and must influence policy. The authors feel that it is generally wise to clear the pelvis where both ovaries are involved to any extent. Implantation of an oestrogen source is easy and effectively bridges the gap of oestrogen deficiency. When this has been necessary and in postoperation discussion the patient is able to appreciate the rationale of what has been done. It is assumed that the surgeon will previously have gone into the question of possibly finding ovarian involvement and its consequences. The surgical options must always be kept open for decision in the operating room and the patient must agree to that so that there are no grounds for future misunderstanding.

There are many centres where a vaginal rather than an abdominal hysterectomy is looked on as the normal or routine method. We do not quarrel with that concept always provided it is not carried to extremes. One has seen an accomplished vaginal surgeon remove a huge fibroid uterus vaginally or perform various procedures on appendages by the same route, but for the average surgeon this can be dangerous. Apart from the dangers of injury to bladder, rectum or ureters haemorrhage can sometimes be difficult to control. If these hazards are avoided or overcome the patient still has to face a convalescence where even limited pelvic blood collections are liable to cause pelvic infection and abscess formation. In the absence of accompanying vaginal vault prolapse it is advisable to limit the use of vaginal hysterectomy to mobile uteri of not more than eight weeks pregnancy size and where there is evidence that the appendages are free and relatively normal.

Vaginal hysterectomy does demand a degree of expertise which only comes with practice and without such experience complications will occur. For this reason it is not an operation for the occasional or inexperienced operator. For the latter the abdominal approach ensures that the various structures and stages of the operation are clearly in his view throughout. The source of any bleeding can be seen immediately and controlled with safety, and unexpected hazards are much less disconcerting than when encountered at the vaginal vault.

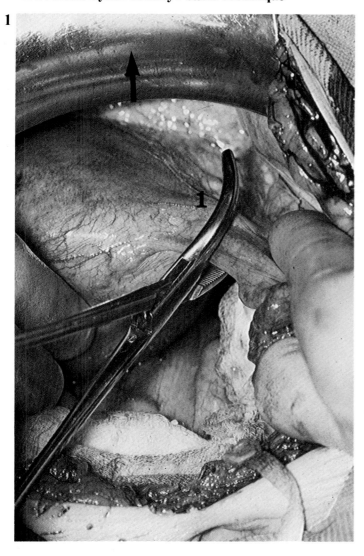

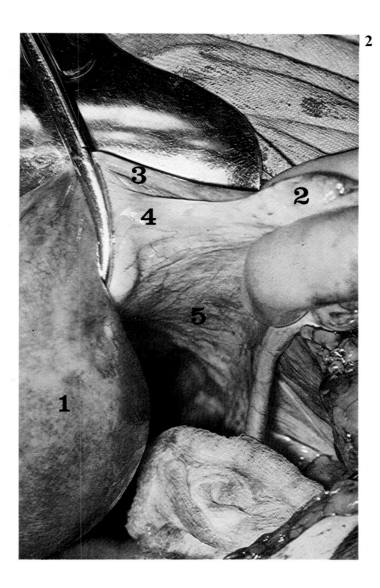

Stage 1: Separation of upper uterine attachments

The abdomen has been opened as described in the previous chapter and a Balfour self-retaining retractor is in place. After a preliminary manual examination of the upper abdominal structures the patient is placed in modified Trendelenburg position so that the omentum and large and small intestines lie in the abdomen outwith the pelvis. This is sometimes facilitated by releasing fine peritoneal attachments lateral to the sigmoid colon with scalpel or scissors; a manoeuvre that also ensures better access to the left infundibulopelvic ligament. A large moist gauze swab is inserted under the upper leaf of the wound in front of the lumbosacral junction to retain the omentum and bowel in the abdomen. The stage is now set to commence the hysterectomy. Before proceeding further the surgeon will take a few moments to examine the uterus and the appendages and particularly the latter. If either ovary is adherent to the side wall of the pelvis or pelvic floor, the ovary is freed with scissors at this stage. Any decision on whether or not ovaries or an ovary is to be removed or retained will probably be taken now.

1 Clamping right broad ligament (1)
The right broad ligament is secured close to the cornu of the uterus with a curved Oschner forceps while the right tube and ovary are held up by the assistant. The attachment of the right round ligament to the uterus is numbered (1). The blade of the Balfour retractor overlies the pubic crest and the arrow indicates the approximate position of the symphysis pubis or midline. The moist retaining swab is seen in the depth of the wound.

2 Clamping right broad ligament (2)
The uterus is held forward and the right ovary laterally to show the structures on the back of the broad ligament. These have been numbered: (1) uterus, (2) ovary, (3) fallopian tube, (4) ovarian ligament, (5) infundibulopelvic ligament.

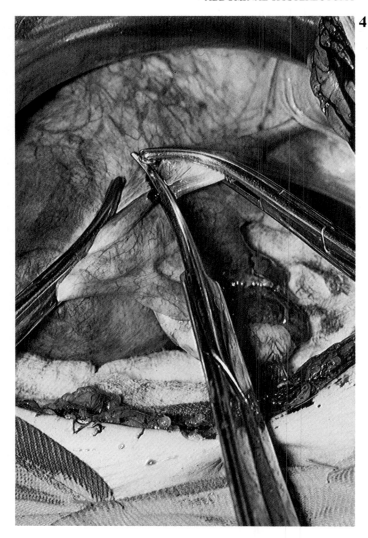

3 Clamping right round ligament

With the Oschner forceps held medially to display the right round ligament a Miles Phillips forceps secures that structure and its overlying peritoneum about its midpoint. A good bite of tissue should be taken to ensure that the ligament and surrounding tissue is firmly in the jaws of the forceps. Unless that is done small vessels accompanying the ligament are not clamped and give irritating bleeding just at the beginning of the operation.

4 Detaching right round ligament

With curved scissors the round ligament is divided between the Oschner and Phillips forceps and the latter fall laterally to expose the interior of the broad ligament. There should be no bleeding if the ligament is firmly grasped; it will be seen that a good cuff of tissue is left on the distal part of the pedicle so that there is no question of it slipping when being ligated.

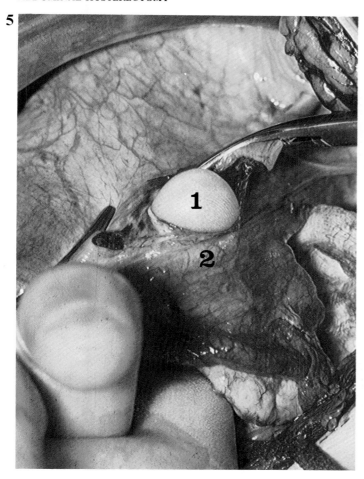

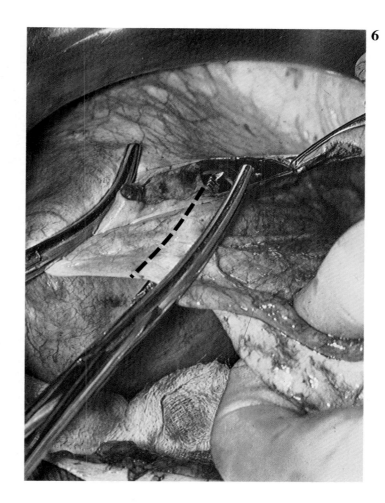

5 Definition of upper right broad ligament

The forefinger (1) is introduced through the posterior layer of the broad ligament opposite the gap in the anterior layer where the round ligament was divided. This opening through the broad ligament defines the upper part of that structure (2).

6 Clamping right broad ligament

The opening in the broad ligament described in Figure 5 is seen. The point of one blade of an Oschner forceps occupies the gap preparatory to closing the jaws of the forceps on the entire pedicle to clamp it firmly. The pedicle will be divided distal to the forceps along the dotted line.

7 Detaching right broad ligament

The broad ligament has been cut across to leave a generous cuff distal to the forceps. The right appendages now fall away laterally.

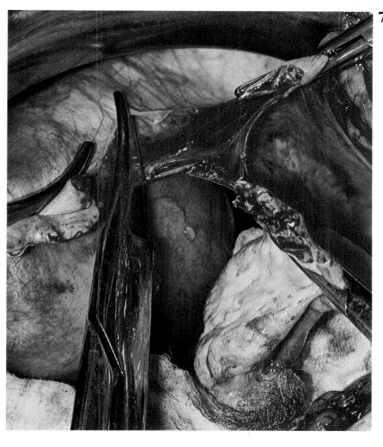

8

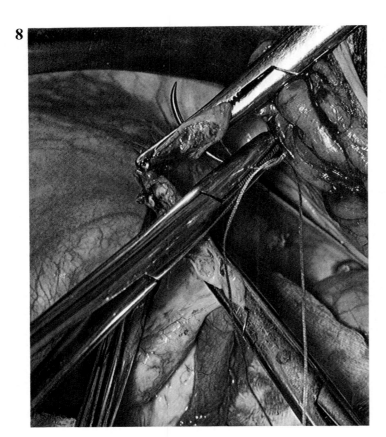

9

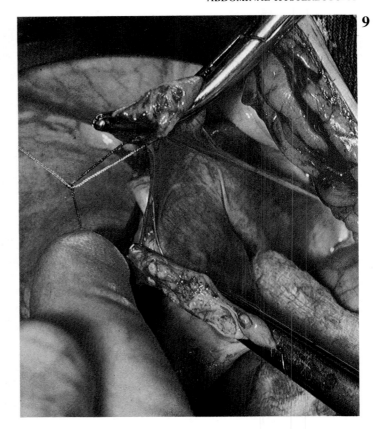

10

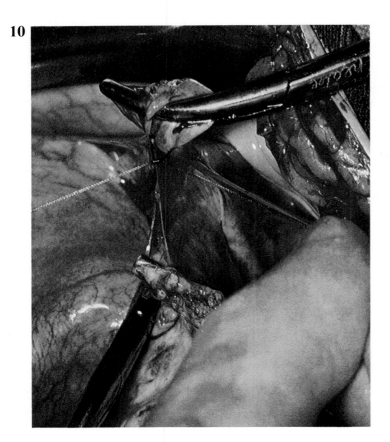

8 to 10 Securing right round ligament pedicle

In Figure 8 the pedicle is transfixed at its midpoint by a curved round-bodied needle carrying a PGA No. 1 suture. In Figure 9 the pedicle is first tied by a single hitch under the toe of the forceps and the suture is then brought back round the pedicle and tied under the heel of the forceps as shown in Figure 10. The first hitch here is a double one to prevent slipping. It is not considered necessary to doubly ligate the round ligament unless there is any doubt about the integrity of the knot.

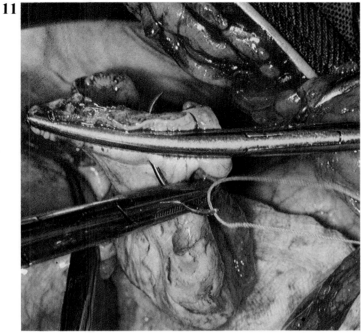

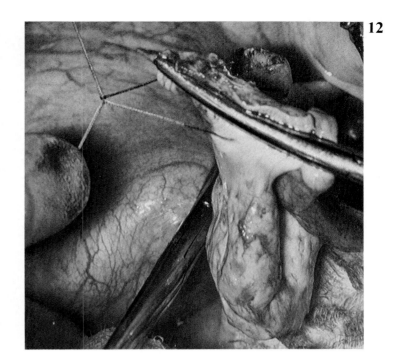

11 to 14 Securing right broad ligament pedicle

In Figures 11, 12 and 13 the same procedure is followed as in Figures 8, 9 and 10, but the pedicle is bulky and it is necessary to ensure that the ligature is secure. In Figure 14 double ligation is being done for added security and is routine for this step.

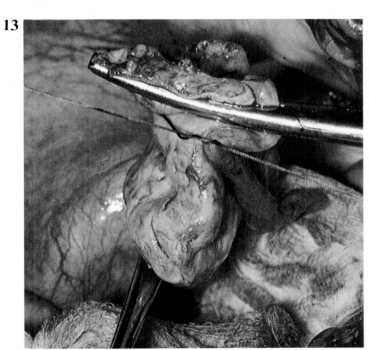

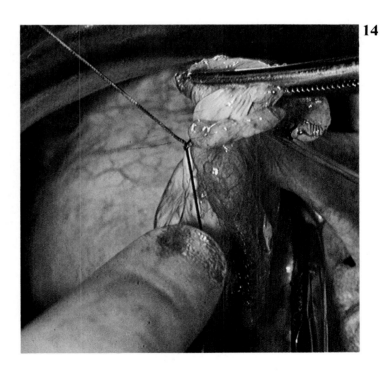

15

16

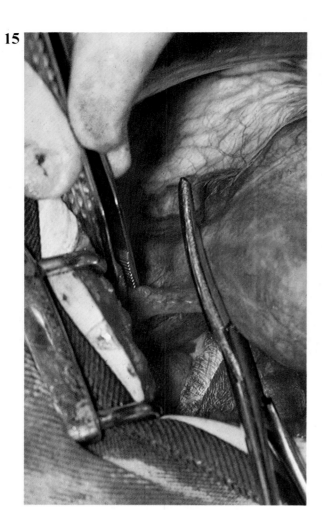

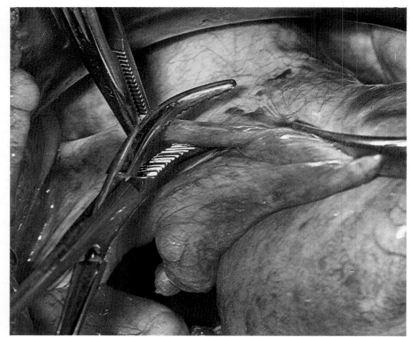

16 Clamping left round ligament
As on the right side.

15 Grasping left broad ligament
As on the right side.

17

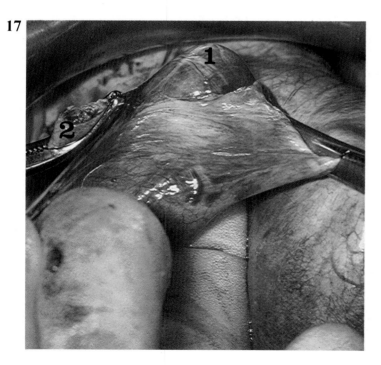

17 Definition of left upper broad ligament
The index finger (1) pushes through the posterior layer of the broad ligament to emerge through the gap anteriorly and define the upper part of the broad ligament. The forceps on the detached (cut) left round ligament are seen (2).

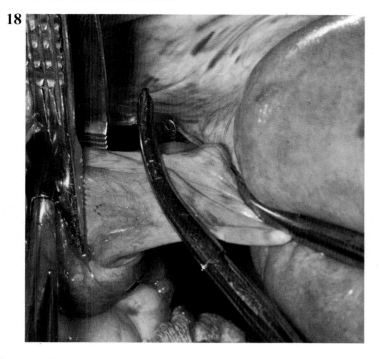

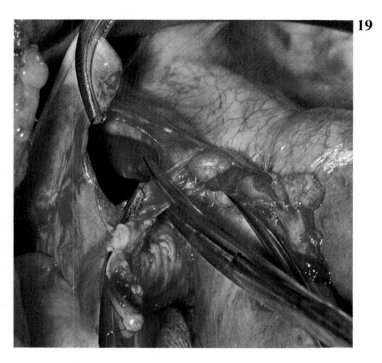

18 Clamping left broad ligament
One blade of the Oschner forceps goes through the gap in the broad ligament and the upper defined pedicle is securely clamped.

19 Detaching left broad ligament pedicle
As on the right side.

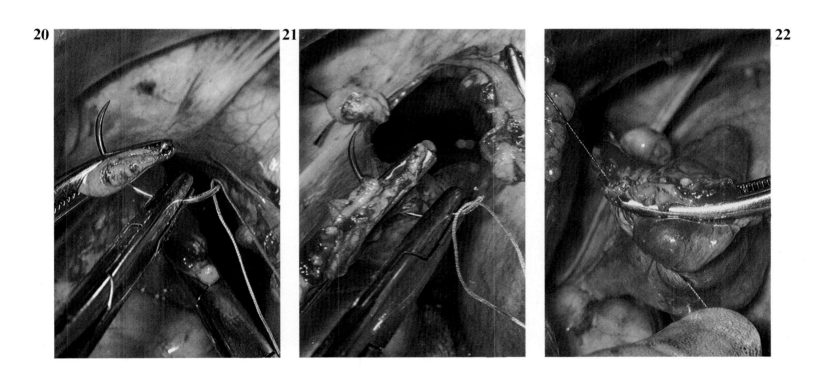

20, 21 and 22 Securing left broad ligament
As on the right side. Note the already ligated left round ligament.

23

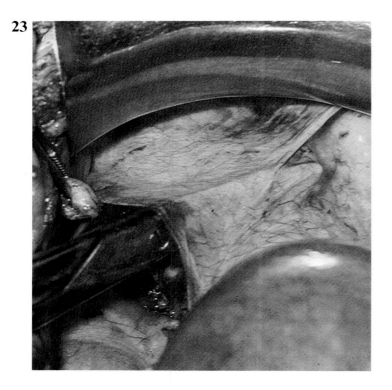

24

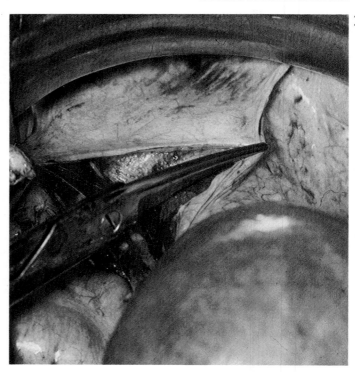

23 Definition of uterovesical pouch (left)
The curved scissors are inserted under the loose peritoneum between the bladder and the uterus on the left side and the blades are opened to form a tunnel ready for incision.

24 Incision of peritoneum of uterovesical pouch (left)
The freed peritoneum is divided with the curved scissors to expose the bladder where it meets the lower uterus anteriorly.

25

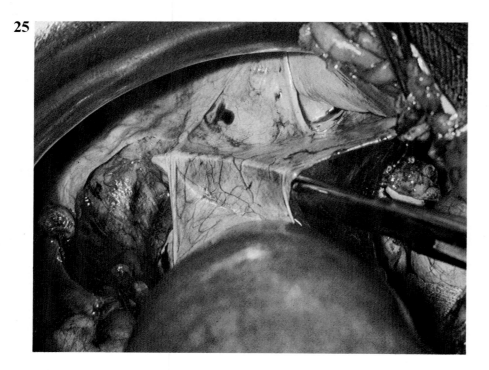

25 Definition of uterovesical pouch (right)
As on the left side.

26

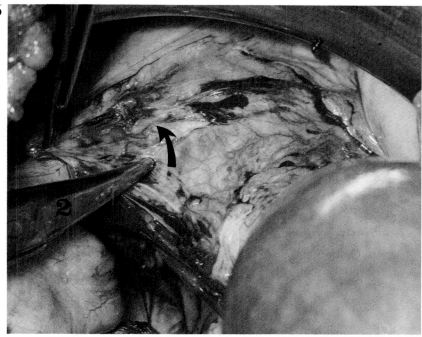

26 Separation of bladder from cervix

Holding the peritoneum covering the bladder with the dissecting forceps (1) the curved scissors (2) are used to separate the bladder off the front of the lower uterus and cervix in the direction of the arrow. We do not favour the method of using a gauze swab on the finger or a swab on a forceps to push the bladder down, because it is liable to result in tearing of a weak bladder wall. If the bladder is held away from the uterus by pulling forward on the peritoneal edge, fine adhesions between the two structures are thrown into relief and can be divided by small snips with the scissors. The blood vessels show up clearly and are easily avoided. Having divided the adhesions the partially open blades of the scissors serve as a very efficient blunt dissector or retractor to push the bladder down off the uterus and cervix.

27

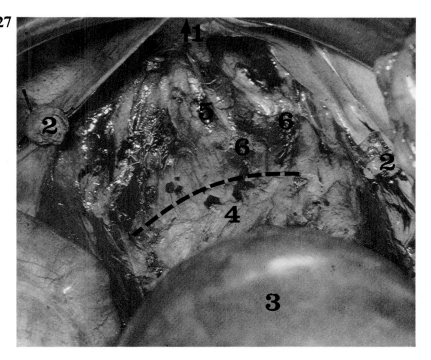

27 Separation of bladder from cervix completed

The pelvic peritoneum is held by forceps (1) to show the superior and part of the posterior aspect of the bladder separated off the front of the uterus. This has been done by sharp dissection taking care to avoid the larger veins and sealing off any small vessels with diathermy. Further separation will in fact be required when the lower uterine attachments have been divided. The various structures are numbered and the broken line indicates the vesicocervical junction: (1) peritoneum held by forceps; (2) round ligament pedicles; (3) fundus uteri; (4) cervix; (5) bladder; (6) diathermy fulguration areas.

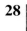

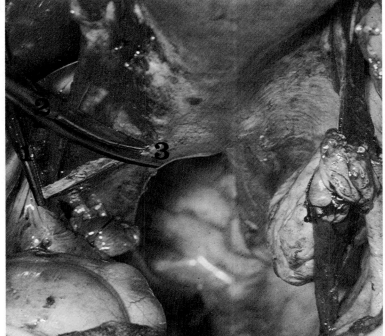

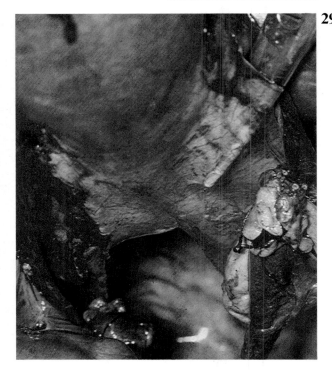

28 to 30 Defining and dividing posterior layer of broad ligaments

To gain access to the uterine vessels it is necessary to open up both leaves of the broad ligament. This has already been done anteriorly and the illustrations show the procedure posteriorly. In Figure 28 the forceps (1) hold the upper edge of the posterior layer on the left side while the curved scissors (2) cut through the peritoneum close to the uterus as far down as the uterosacral ligament (3). In Figure 29 preparation is made to do the same on the right side by raising the peritoneum with the scissors to make a tunnel. In Figure 30 the incision is made as on the left side. The number (4) indicates the ligated broad ligaments. Arrows indicate the uterine arteries.

31

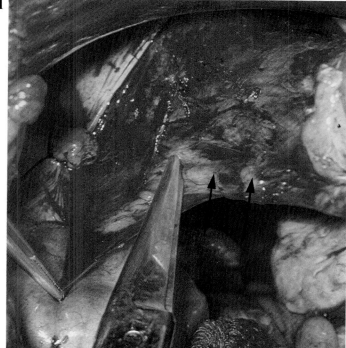

32

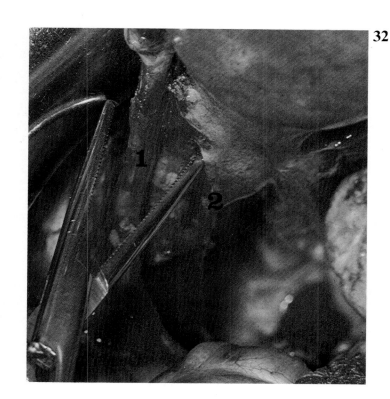

31 Defining left uterine pedicle

With the broad ligament opened up there is free access to the uterine vessels and these are carefully stripped free of loose fat and light adhesions by gentle snips with the scissors. The loose tissues fall back in a very gratifying manner to expose the arteries and veins (arrowed). Readers are strongly advised not to adopt the dangerous practice of stripping back the tissues with a gauze swab, because it tears veins and causes bleeding.

32 and 33 Clamping left uterine pedicle

The vessels have been clearly isolated in Figure 32 (1) and a straight Oschner forceps is in process of being applied. The point of the posterior limb of the forceps is placed against the uterus just above the attachment of the uterosacral ligament (2) and the jaws closed so that the line of the forceps is nearly at right angles to the vertical axis of the uterus. In Figure 33 this angle is shown and also confirms that the anterior limb of the forceps is close in on the uterus (3) so that no branches of the artery are missed. The outline of the ectocervix is marked by a broken line.

33

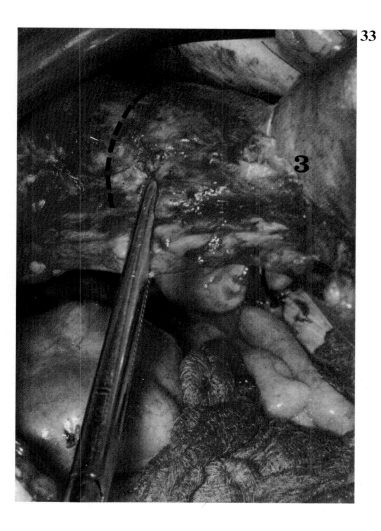

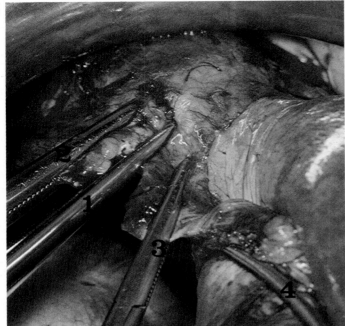

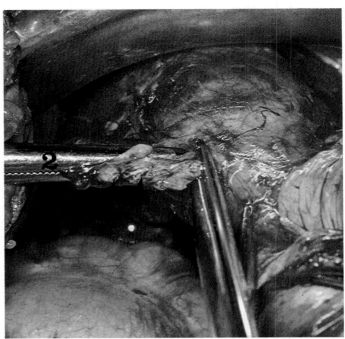

34 to 36 Detachment of left uterine pedicle

In Figure 34 straight scissors (1) divide the uterine pedicle between the straight Oschner forceps just applied (2) and small Spencer Wells forceps applied to prevent back flow of blood from the uterine body (3). The cut is made parallel to the larger forceps leaving a good cuff of tissue and is carried right up to the uterine wall. The number 4 indicates the holding forceps on the left cornu of the uterus. In Figure 35 the uterine pedicle is further freed from the uterus by making a short cut at right angles to the first just beyond the point of the forceps (2). Note the cut ends of the uterine arteries in the pedicle (arrowed). In Figure 36 the forceps (2) are used as a

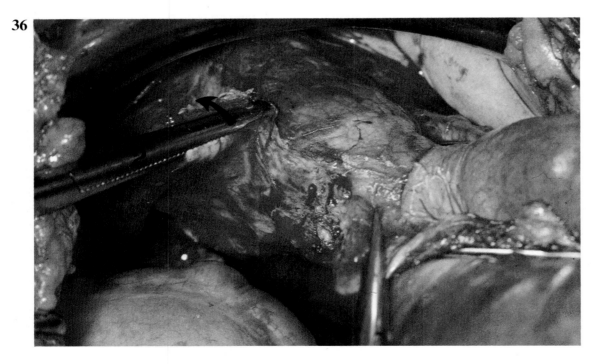

lever to strip the pedicle off the side of the uterus by a controlled rolling and pushing movement in the direction of the arrow. The uterine pedicle with its vessels is now quite free and can be safely tied without fear of it slipping from the ligature.

37

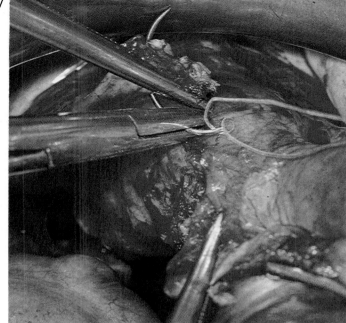

38

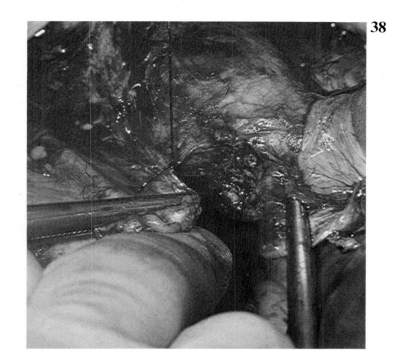

37 to 40 Ligation of left uterine pedicle

The various steps of transfixion at the midpoint, ligation and double ligation have already been described on page 48 and are carried out at this stage. PGA No. 1 suture on a round-bodied needle is used and care is taken to place a secure ligature. This is obviously most important.

39

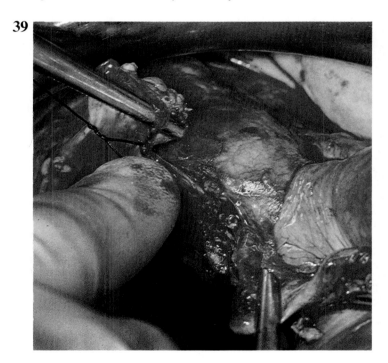

40

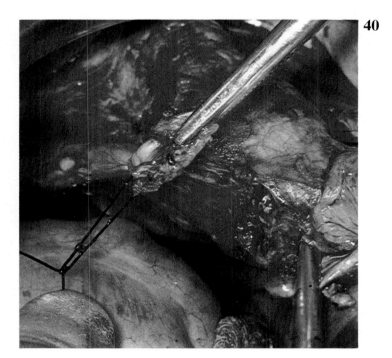

41

42

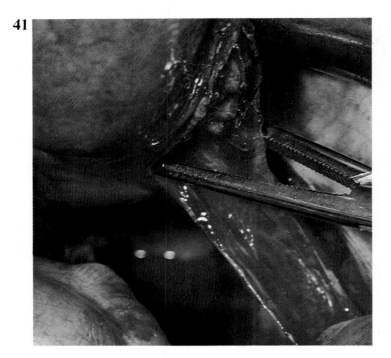

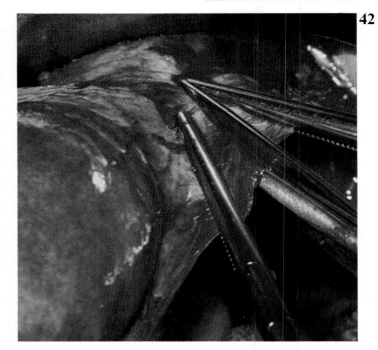

41 and 42 Clamping and detaching right uterine pedicle
As on the left side. Note the angle at which the pedicle is
clamped and cut.

43

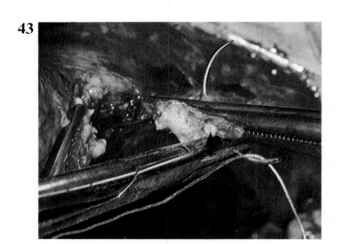

43 and 44 Ligation of right uterine pedicle
As on the left side. Note the importance of having freed or
defined the pedicle for ligation. The uterine arteries are again
arrowed.

44

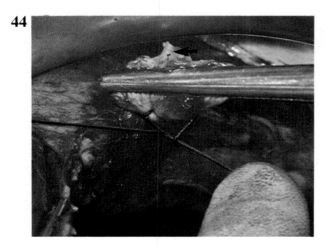

Stage 3: Dividing lower uterine attachments

45

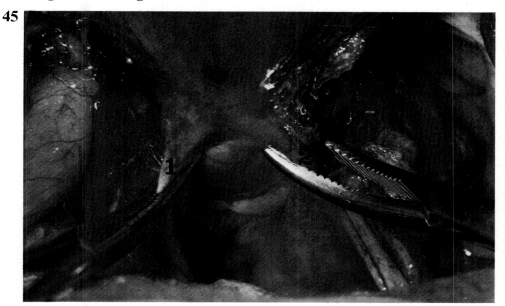

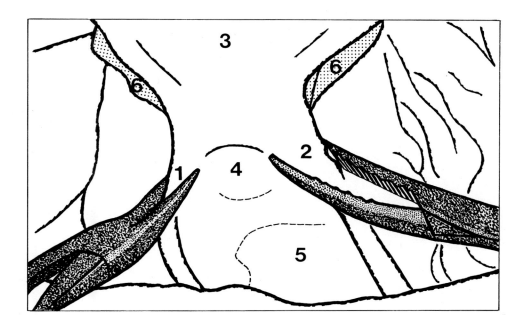

With the uterine vessels secured, the uterus is held up and forwards but it is still firmly attached to the floor of the pelvis by the uterosacral ligaments; the next step is to detach these from the uterus. Once that has been done, the uterus can be lifted up to give access to the vaginal angles which contain the transverse cervical or cardinal ligaments.

45 Clamping uterosacral ligaments

In the illustration the left uterosacral ligament has been secured (1) and the right is in the process of being clamped (2). The site is just clear of the bulk of the uterus and a good firm bite of tissue is taken so that any accompanying vessels are not excluded. The main sutures are numbered on the accompanying diagram.

1 Left uterosacral ligament
2 Right uterosacral ligament
3 Uterus
4 Cervix
5 Rectum
6 Ligated uterine pedicles

46

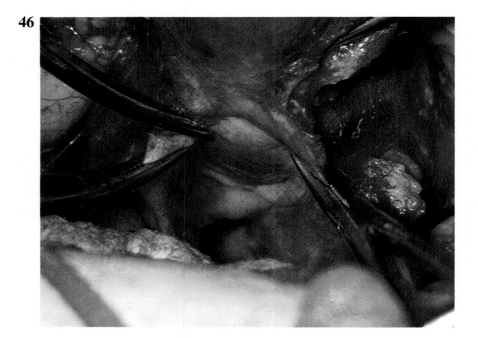

46 Detaching uterosacral ligaments

The left uterosacral ligament is detached from the uterus with scissors cutting distal to the holding forceps and the same is then done on the other side.

47

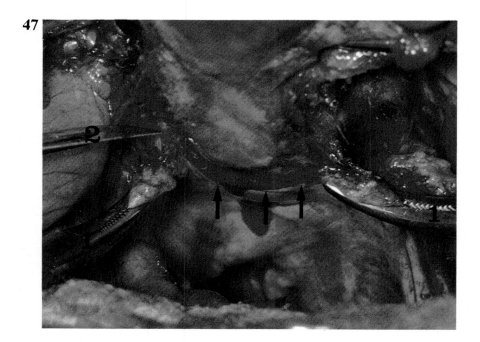

47 Freeing the uterus posteriorly

Both uterosacral ligaments have been separated off the uterus and are held in the forceps (1). The scalpel (2) has completed a stroke across the posterior aspect of the cervix at the level of its inferior border to divide the peritoneum (arrowed) where it is attached to the posterior aspect of the cervix and also to divide any superficial fibrous tissue which is still anchoring the uterus. Immediately this is done, the uterus can be lifted up from the pelvic floor and the uterosacral ligaments fall back free of it as shown in Figure 51 (opposite).

48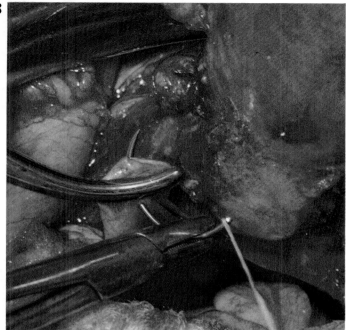

49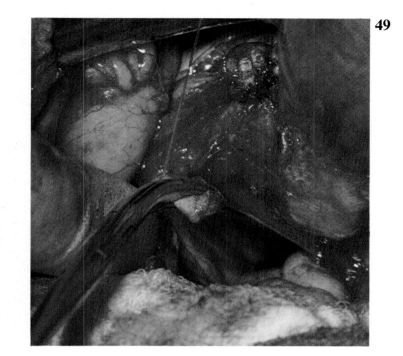

48 to 51 Ligation of uterosacral ligaments

In Figure 48 the left ligament is being transfixed and in Figure 49 tied. The right ligament is being ligated in Figure 50 and in Figure 51 the posterior aspect of the uterus is shown completely freed. The pedicles are numbered thus: (1) uterine, (2) broad ligament, (3) uterosacral, and (4) round ligament.

50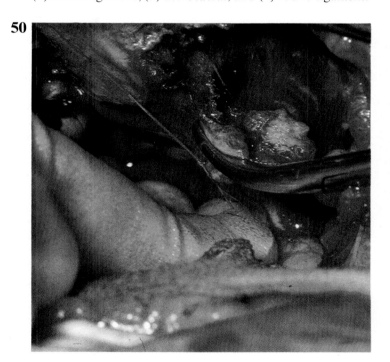

51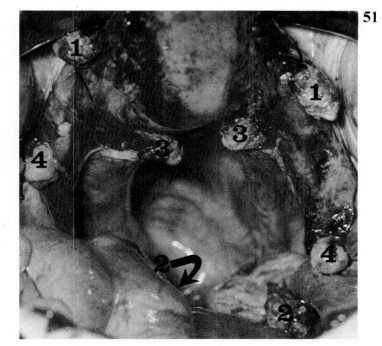

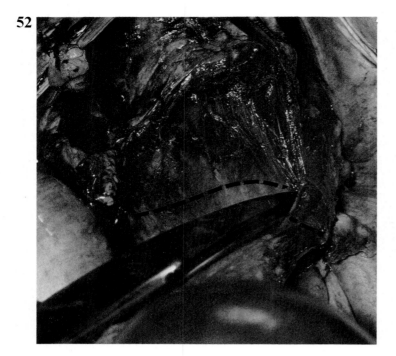

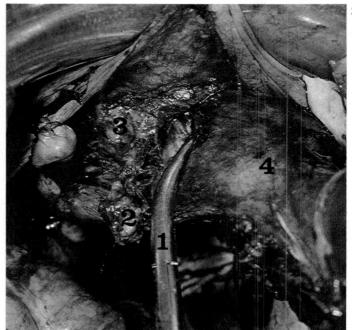

52 Separation of bladder from uterus

As indicated previously it is necessary to further separate the bladder from the anterior aspect of the cervix, but this is difficult until the uterosacral ligaments have been cut so that the uterus can be lifted up to give deeper access anteriorly. In the illustration the curved scissors are used to free the bladder by pushing with the closed blades and making small snips until an adequate depth has been reached. The line of the bladder attachment is indicated by the broken line.

53 and 54 Clamping left vaginal angle

The operator holds up the uterus in one hand and checks between the forefinger and thumb of the other that the vagina can be entered below the level of the cervix (4). A curved Oschner forceps (1) is then applied medial to and clear of the ligated uterine pedicle (2). It is also clear of the bladder edge anteriorly (3) and when closed includes the whole vaginal angle and the medial part of the cardinal ligament. The anterior placement and view is shown on Figure 53 and the posterior view in Figure 54. The general outline of the cervix can be seen in both (4).

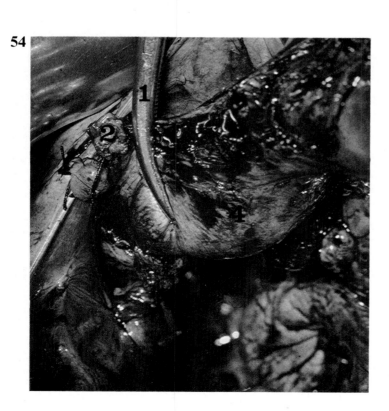

55

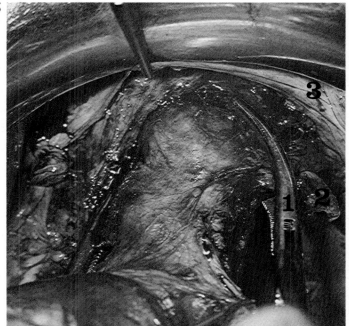

56

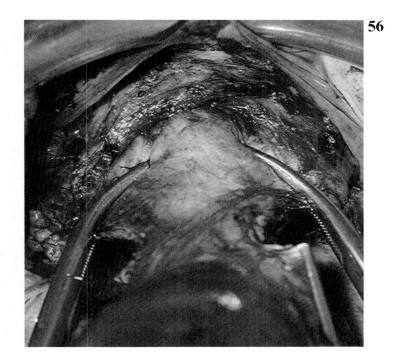

55 to 57 Securing both vaginal angles

In Figure 55 the right vaginal angle is clamped as on the other side (1) and is seen to be clear of the uterine pedicle (2) and the bladder (3). The outline of the cervix is again clear. In Figure 56 a direct anterior view shows the placement of the clamps; in Figure 57 the uterus is lifted forwards to show the posterior aspect. The general outline of the cervix (4) is obvious.

57

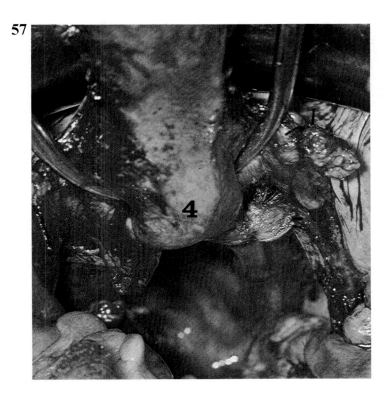

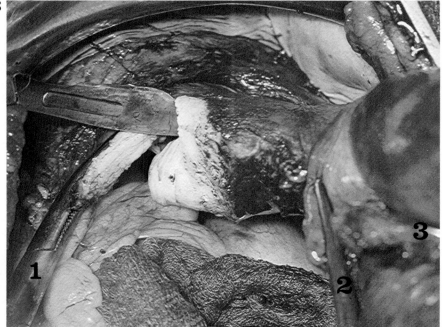

58 Incision into vaginal vault (left)

With the scalpel, the angle of the vagina is entered by cutting at a distance of 0.5 cm beyond the forceps (1). The vaginal edge curls back to show the cavity as air is audibly drawn in. Forceps (2) are on the uterine end of the vascular pedicle to prevent backflow and forceps (3) are on the broad ligament near the cornu of the uterus.

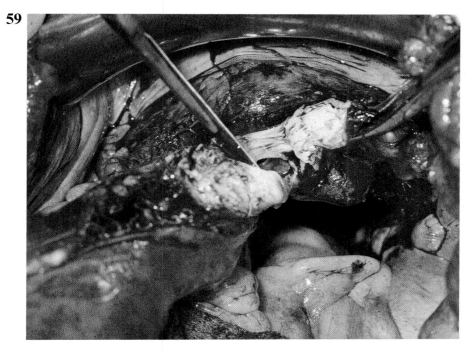

59 Incision into vaginal vault (right)

The same manoeuvre is carried out on the opposite side; as a result the uterus is now attached to the vagina only by an anterior and posterior band of tissue.

60

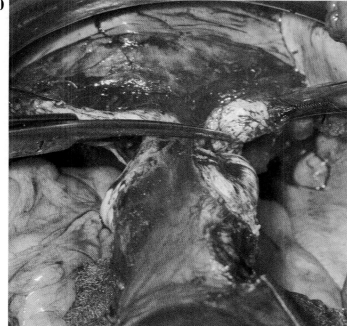

61

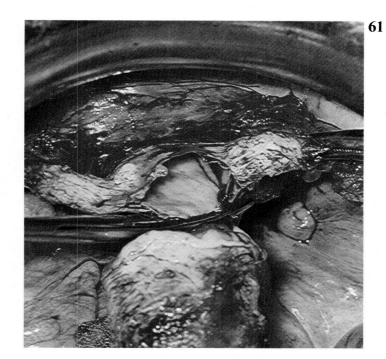

60 to 62 Separation of uterus from vagina

In Figure 60 the curved scissors are used to divide across the anterior vaginal wall where the uterus is attached. The line of the incision is kept well clear of the cervix to avoid the thickened tissue in that area and cuts through the vaginal wall only. In Figure 61 the posterior vaginal wall is similarly divided and again keeping well clear of the cervix. The uterus is now free. In Figure 62 the vaginal vault is seen displayed and open with the forceps on the vaginal angles still in place (1). The posterior wall is now held by a Littlewood's forceps (2).

62

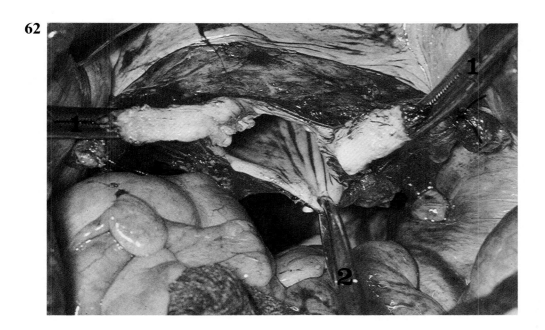

Stage 5: Reconstruction of vaginal vault

With the uterus removed and the vaginal vault open, the next stage is to ensure a closure which will make the vault at least as firm as previously. This is aided by attaching the ends of the uterosacral ligaments to the vault during closure; the method is described below. We do not generally favour the use of the round ligaments for that purpose as it seems that they are thereby put under an unnatural tension; in any case they do not contain sufficient fibrous or muscular tissue to exert any supportive effect at such a disadvantageous angle. Some surgeons prefer to leave the vault open in vascular or infected cases to ensure adequate drainage. Others consistently leave the vault open and believe that this is the correct procedure in all cases. We disagree with the latter but believe the former group are acting logically in special cases. If the vault is left open steps must be taken to prevent bleeding from the cut edge; this is generally effected by placing a blanket stitch all round the edge of the vault, sufficiently tight to control bleeding or oozing. The completed stitch has the effect of drawing the vault together in a purse-string fashion so that the opening becomes quite small. When covered over on the inner aspect by the closed peritoneum there is very little chance of herniation taking place through it. This question is referred to again on page 68.

63

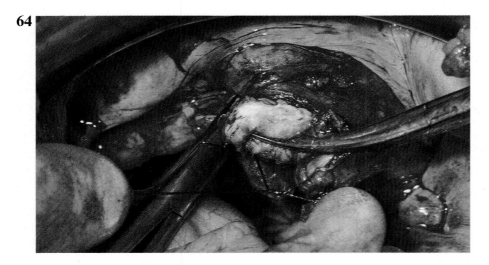

63 and 64 Ligation of right vaginal angle

A cutting needle carrying a PGA No. 1 suture pierces each vaginal wall in turn, proximal and just medial to the point of the forceps, so that when tied it will include all the vessels at the angle. The ligature is not tied round the toe of the forceps but only under its heel and kept as far proximal as possible to avoid any tendency to slip off. This is illustrated in Figure 64 where the first double hitch is being run up. There is no question of attempting a double ligation because it is not possible to bring the suture under the point of the forceps. The stitch should be carefully and strongly tied. If there is any doubt about its security, then the use of a needle-mounted suture with repetition of the process is suggested.

64

65

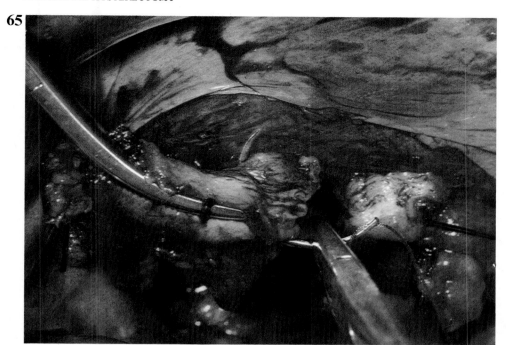

65 Ligation of left vaginal angle

As on right side. This photograph shows how bulky the
pedicle can be, especially if the cardinal ligament has been the
site of previous inflammatory, traumatic or endometriotic
involvement.

66

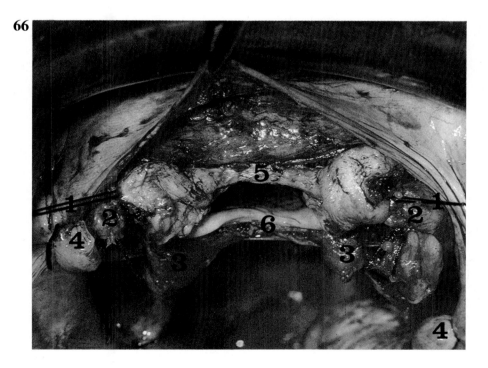

66 Vaginal vault with angles secured

The two angles are held laterally by the uncut sutures (1). The
uterine pedicles (2), the uterosacral ligaments (3), the round
ligaments (4), the anterior vaginal wall (5) and the posterior
vaginal wall (6) are shown.

Stage 6: Closure of vaginal vault to incorporate uterosacral ligaments

With the angles of the vaginal vault closed and held laterally it remains to close the vaginal opening medially; this step is effected by using three mattress sutures. The two lateral sutures transfix and include the uterosacral pedicle of its own side which is thereby attached to the posterior aspect of the suture line as is shown in the serial photographs. The central mattress suture includes only the two vaginal walls. The reader will realise that if the vault is left open the uterosacral ligaments lose almost all their supportive function, with an increased likelihood of subsequent enterocele or even vault prolapse. A raw granulation area persists at the vault of the vagina for several weeks and causes a vaginal discharge. For these reasons the authors routinely close the vault, although agreeing that in particular circumstances it might be very reasonable to leave it open.

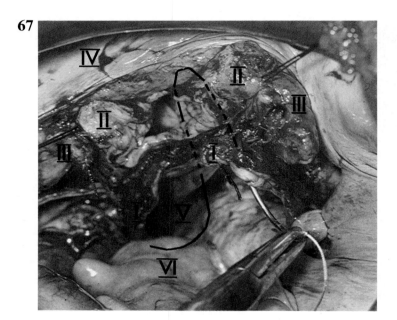

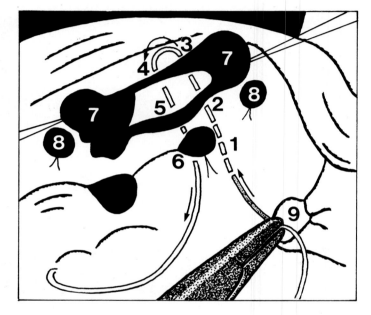

67 Closure of vaginal vault (right) (1)

This is the first step in the procedure and shows the needle with a PGA No. 1 suture picking up the right uterosacral pedicle before transfixing the vaginal edges and returning to pierce the pedicle again before being tied off. The dotted line indicates the line taken by the suture. In the diagram this line is repeated and the structures incorporated in the stitch are numbered in sequence 1 to 6.

The line taken by the suture is shown on the diagram. The main structures and pedicles are denoted by roman numerals thus: (I) uterosacral pedicles; (II) vaginal angles; (III) uterine pedicles; (IV) bladder; (V) pouch of Douglas; (VI) rectum.

1 Right uterosacral ligament
2 Posterior vaginal wall
3 Anterior vaginal wall
4 Anterior vaginal wall
5 Posterior vaginal wall
6 Right uterosacral ligament
Other structures seen are:
7 Ligated vaginal angles
8 Ligated uterine vessels
9 Right round ligament ligated

68 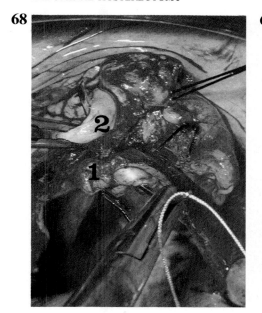 **69** 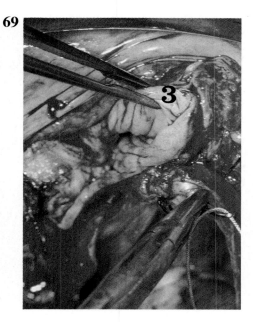 **70**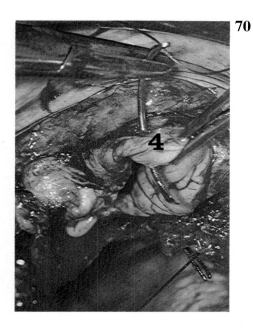

68 to 73 Closure of vaginal vault (right) (2)

The route taken by the suture to complete the mattress suture on the right side is shown progressively. In Figure 68 the stitch already through the uterosacral ligament (1) pierces the posterior vaginal wall (2), and in Figure 69 the anterior vaginal wall (3). In Figure 70 it returns through the anterior vaginal wall (4) and in Figure 71 the posterior vaginal wall (5). In Figure 72 it again picks up the uterosacral ligament in such a way as to encircle it when tied (6). Figure 73 shows the stitch being tied.

71 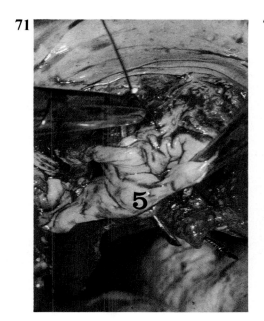 **72** 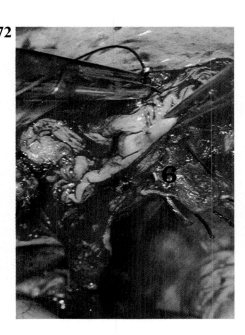 **73**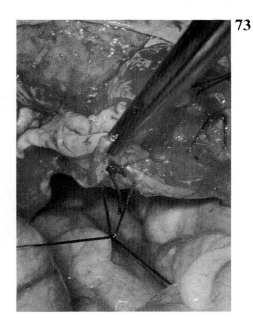

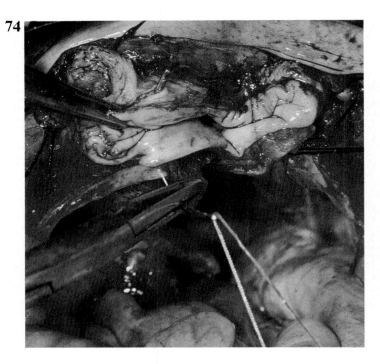

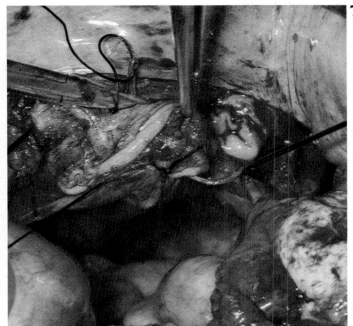

74 to 76 Closure of vaginal vault (left)

The same procedure is shown in three stages. Figure 74 shows the three bites taken by the needle on the outward journey and Figure 75 the same in reverse on the return journey, and the stitch is being tied to incorporate the uterosacral pedicle in Figure 76.

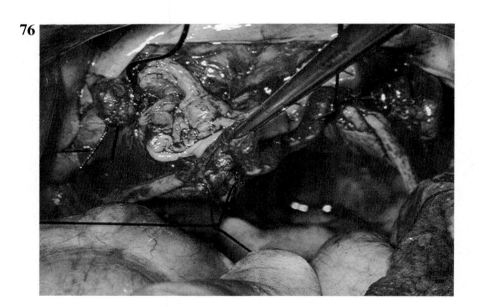

77

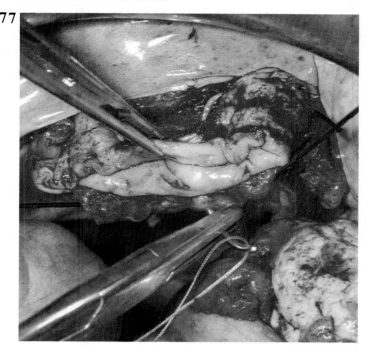

78

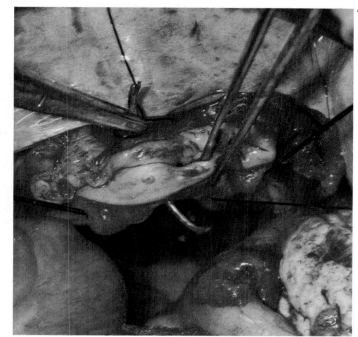

77 to 79 Closing vaginal vault centrally

A simple mattress suture closes the vault as shown and traverses vaginal wall tissue only. Figure 77 shows the outward journey, Figure 78 the return journey and Figure 79 ligation. In some cases where the vault is narrow a simple through-and-through stitch may suffice; if the vault is very wide an additional mattress suture may be required.

79

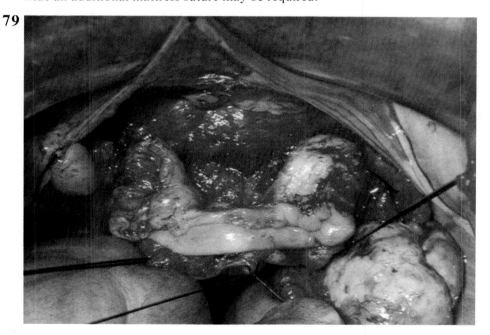

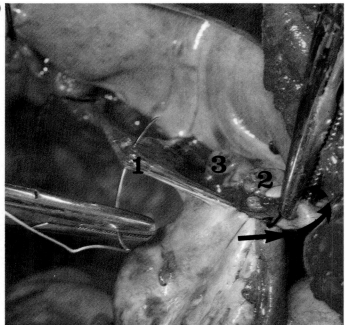

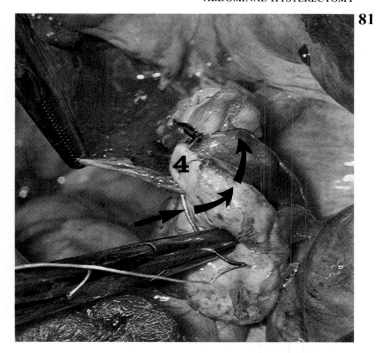

At this stage the surgeon ensures that there is no bleeding or oozing from the operation field and prepares to close the peritoneum across the pelvic floor. Normally there is no question of draining the area but if circumstances arose where that was thought necessary, it would be at this stage that one would place a small polythene suction drain of the Redivac type across the vault of the vagina. This would lie extraperitoneally with the end brought through the skin lateral to the incision. Two such drains are often used, one emerging on each side.

In a routine closure the PGA No. 00 suture commences on the right side where it approximates the anterior and posterior peritoneal edges in such a way as to cover over the ligated round and broad ligament pedicles. It then runs across the pelvic floor approximating the peritoneal leaves in an over-and-over stitch to end by burying the same pedicles on the opposite side in the same fashion. As the stitch crosses the vault of the vagina, the authors consider it good practice to attach the edges of the peritoneum to the vaginal margins and so eliminate dead space in the depth of the wound, i.e. at the vaginal vault.

80 Closure of pelvic peritoneum (1)
The needle commences by transfixing the posterior edge of the peritoneum (1) preparatory to travelling laterally (in the direction of the curved arrow) round the broad ligament pedicle (2) (which is shown held in forceps) and the round ligament pedicle (3). This manoeuvre forms a partial purse-string suture which will bury the pedicles.

81 Closure of pelvic peritoneum (2)
The needle with its transfixed peritoneum now picks up the ovarian ligament (4) and already the concept of the inverting suture is appreciated.

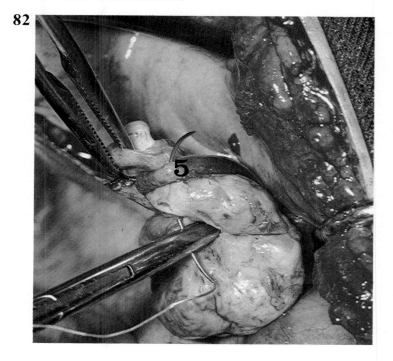

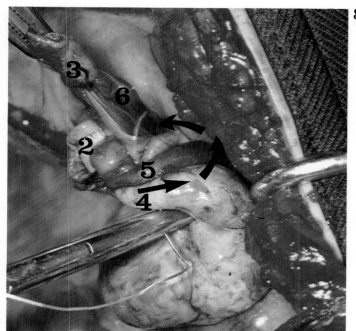

82 to 84 Closure of pelvic peritoneum (3)

The needle has already picked up the fallopian tube (5) in Figure 82 and is about to transfix the anterior layer of peritoneum overlying the round ligament at point (6) in

Figure 83. Both the broad ligament pedicle (2) and the round ligament pedicle (3) will now be within the stitch. In Figure 84 this stitch is tied and the pedicles are receding under the peritoneal edge.

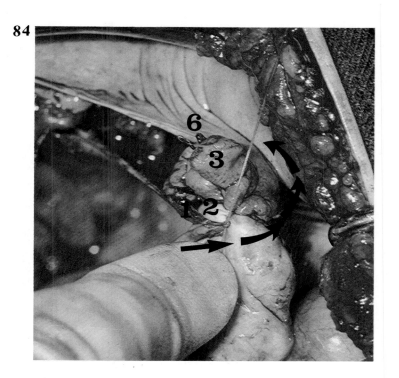

85

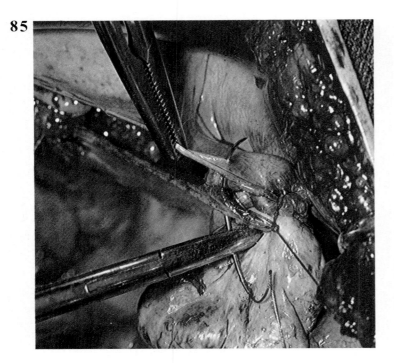

86

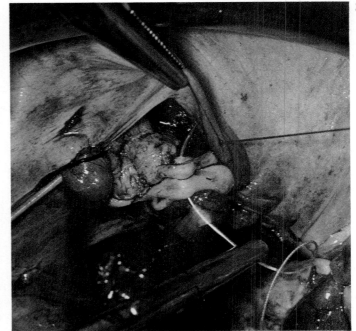

85 to 88 Closure of pelvic peritoneum (4)

In Figure 85 the stitch is commencing its journey across the pelvic floor. In Figure 86 the manner of attaching the leaves of the peritoneum to the vaginal vault is shown, and in Figure 87 the stitch is tied off after having completed a similar type of purse-string procedure to bury the broad and round ligament pedicles on the left side. Figure 88 shows the closed pelvic peritoneum.

87

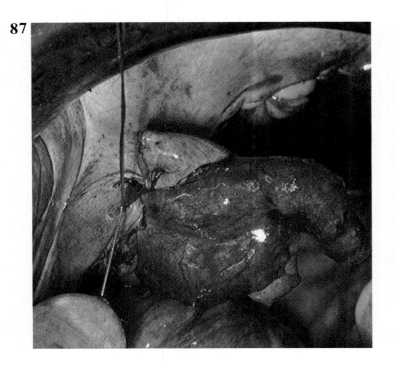

88

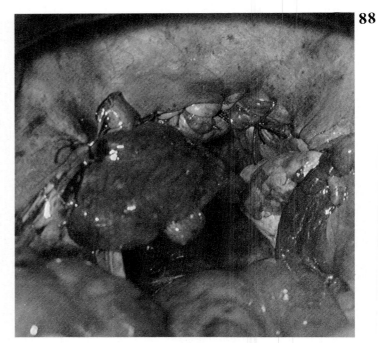

Conditions demanding modification of basic hysterectomy technique: broad ligament fibroid

When a fibroid or mass of fibroids extends laterally between the leaves of the broad ligament they can create difficulties during hysterectomy; the larger the mass the greater the problem. Sometimes the uterus is found perched on top of a large fibroid mass which underlies the peritoneum and occupies most of the pelvic space. Such fibroids develop from the lower part of the body of the uterus rather than from the cervix and are initially subserous. They extend laterally as they grow anteriorly or posteriorly to the uterine vessels and raise the pelvic peritoneum on their surface; the extent to which it is raised depends on the size of the fibroid. The ureter is adherent to the extraperitoneal surface and is carried up and laterally so that in extreme cases it lies laterally but also on top of the fibroid. In hysterectomy, and unless the surgeon knows how to deal with the problem, there is a real risk of ureteric damage.

The hysterectomy should commence on the same side as the fibroid, opening up the broad ligament in the usual way by detaching the round ligament and the upper broad ligament and keeping close to the side of the uterus. The anterior and posterior layers of the broad ligament are further opened up in a sagittal plane and the leaves are easily separated laterally off the fibroid mass. This is done by blunt dissection and keeping a look out for the ureter attached to the under surface of the peritoneum. It is usually easy to recognise and when found is under-run with a tape or held in a ureteric forceps. It can then be dissected with its peritoneal attachments quite clear of the fibroid. This dissection is carried as far anteriorly as the ureteric tunnel and posteriorly to the ovarian fossa. The surgeon's fingers are then inserted under the fibroid; by blunt dissection it is nearly always possible to lift the mass upwards and medially off the pelvic floor and so display the uterine vessels. These are seen underneath and medially and having become accessible allow for safe hysterectomy.

The unaffected side of the uterus is now detached from its upper attachments and hysterectomy is straightforward.

On occasion the fibroid cannot be elevated in this way because it is essentially intramural. In such circumstances the best procedure is to make a short deep incision in the coronal plane keeping clear of the uterine vessels and cut down into the capsule of the fibroid to expose myomatous tissue. The fibroid tissue is grasped with a volsellum or a series of Littlewood's forceps and enucleated while it is held up on the stretch. A deep figure of eight haemostatic suture will control any bleeding from the cavity and the anatomy of the lower uterus is immediately restored. Hysterectomy becomes a safe and straightforward procedure.

Stage 1: Separation of upper uterine supports

1 General view to show right broad ligament fibroid
The appearance is typical, with one fibroid deep in the right broad ligament (1), and the round ligament running over it (2). There is another fibroid on the anterior aspect of the uterus (3). A curved Oschner forceps holds the broad ligament (4) displaying the ovary (5) and the fallopian tube (6) while the displaced right ureter can be seen laterally under the peritoneum (arrowed).

2 Clamping right round ligament
The hysterectomy commences on the affected side by clamping the round ligament between forceps (1) and (2), close to the uterus. Forceps (4) on the broad ligament are still visible.

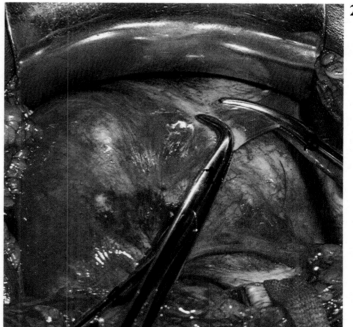

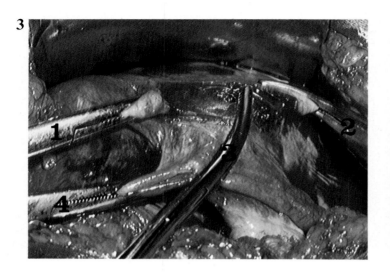

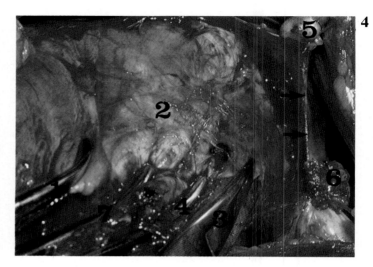

3 Clamping right upper broad ligament

With the round ligament divided between forceps (1) and (2) a curved Oschner forceps clamps the upper broad ligament (3) just lateral and close to the holding forceps (4).

4 Broad ligament opened: fibroid exposed

The peritoneum (arrowed) is pulled laterally to expose the upper aspect of the fibroid (2); the scissors commencing lateral blunt dissection (3). The ligated round ligament (5) and broad ligament (6) are seen with the original forceps (1) and (4) on their uterine cut ends respectively. An extra forceps has been applied to the broad ligament between forceps (4) and the uterus to give a stronger hold when elevating the uterus and the attached fibroid. It is numbered (7).

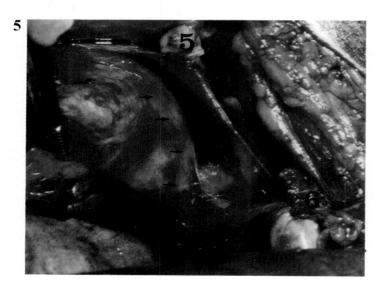

5 Lateral dissection of peritoneum

The peritoneum has been lifted upwards and laterally between the round ligament (5) and the broad ligament (6) leaving the right ureter (arrowed) on the surface and lightly attached to the fibroid.

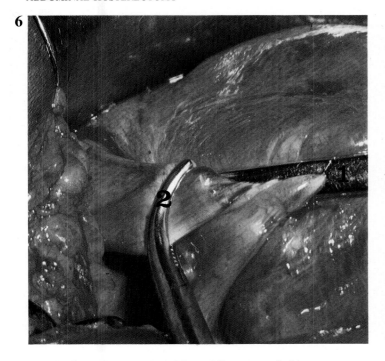

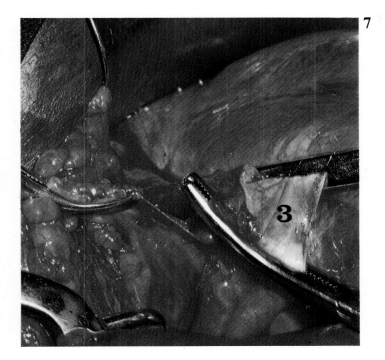

6 to 8 Clamping round and broad ligaments (left)

The uterine attachment of the broad ligament is held in forceps (1) while the round ligament is clamped (2) in Figure 6 and the broad ligament (3) in Figure 7. Both ligaments have been detached from the uterus in Figure 8.

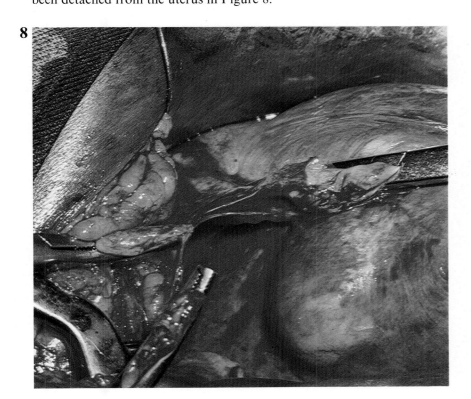

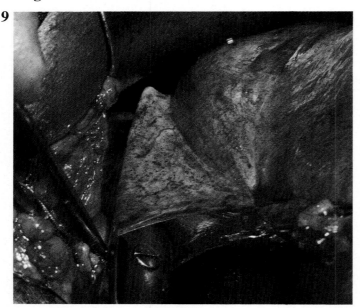

9 Definition of right ureter (1)
Returning to the right side of the uterus the peritoneum of the uterovesical pouch is defined with the scissors before opening it up to give access anteriorly.

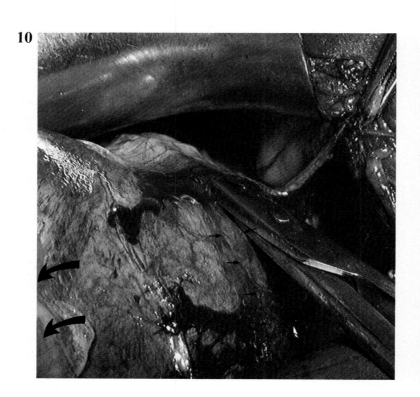

10 Definition of right ureter (2)
Dissection of the peritoneum from the fibroid continues laterally and further displays the ureter (small arrows). The uterus and its attached fibroid are meantime pulled medially and upwards from the pelvic floor. The surgeon's fingers can be seen pulling the uterus in the direction of the arrows.

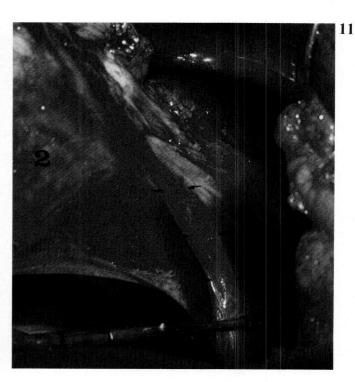

11 Definition of right ureter (3)
The ureter (small arrows) and held in Allis' forceps (1) is being pushed laterally off the fibroid (2) which is strongly retracted medially with forceps.

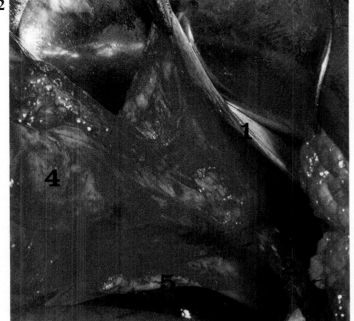

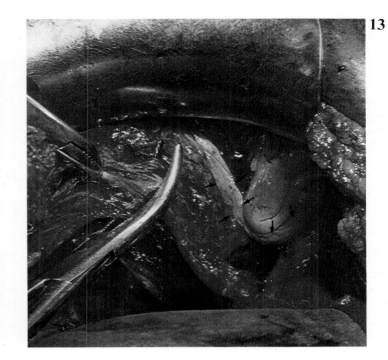

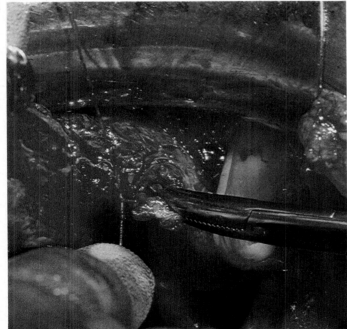

12 Definition of uterine vessels (right)

With the ureter further encouraged to the right and with the fibroid pulled medially by forceps the leash of uterine vessels stands out clearly. Note that the lower part of the posterior leaf of the broad ligament persists and will now be divided. The numbers and overlays indicate the various structures: peritoneal edge (1); ureter outline (2); tape on ureter (3); fibroid (4); uncut posterior broad ligament (5).

13 and 14 Securing uterine vessels (right)

With the ureter clearly visible (small arrows) the uterine pedicle is safely clamped sufficiently close to the uterus to avoid any distortion of the ureter when tied and with a sufficient cuff to prevent slipping.

Stage 4: Completion of hysterectomy

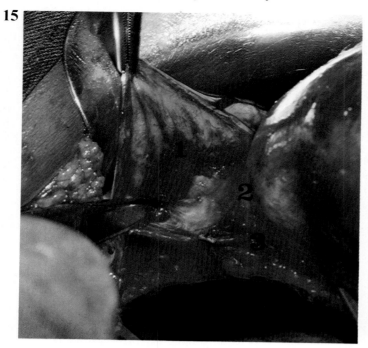

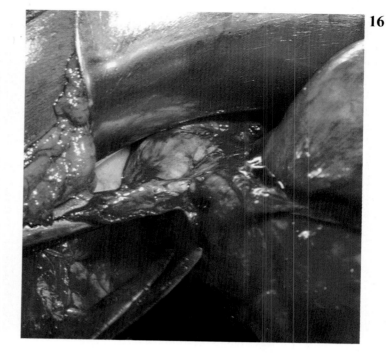

15 to 18 Defining and detaching lower uterine attachments (left)

In Figure 15 the bladder (1) is further separated by sharp scissors dissection from the front of the cervix (2) to expose the uterine vessels (3). In Figure 16 the clamped uterine vessels have just been detached and in Figure 17 ligated. Figure 18 shows the angle of the vagina secured by forceps (4) medial to the ligated uterine pedicle and clear of the bladder which is being held back by dissecting forceps (5). The same procedure is then carried out on the right side.

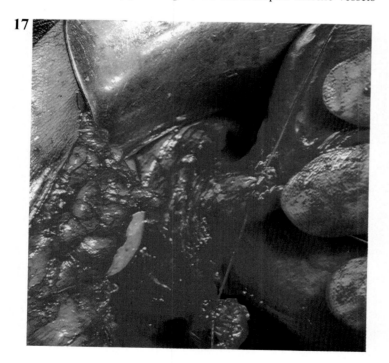

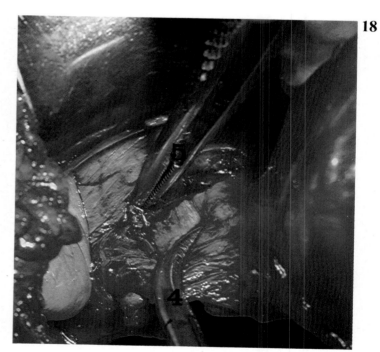

19

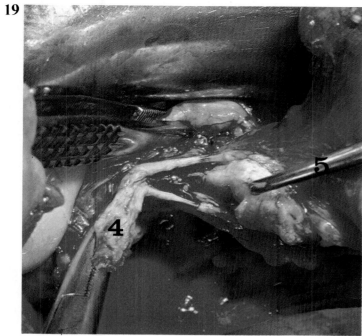

19 and 20 Removing uterus

In Figure 19 the vaginal vault is opened medial to the forceps on the angle (4) and the cervix is picked up by Littlewood's forceps (5). In Figure 20 the right side has similarly been opened and the uterus removed to show the open vaginal cavity (6) ready for transverse closure.

20

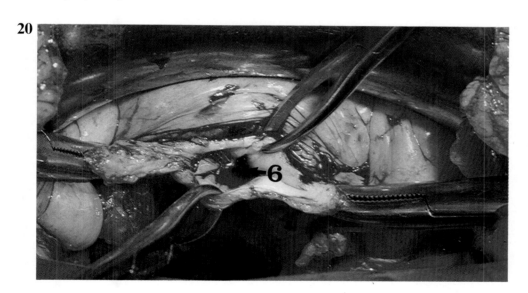

21

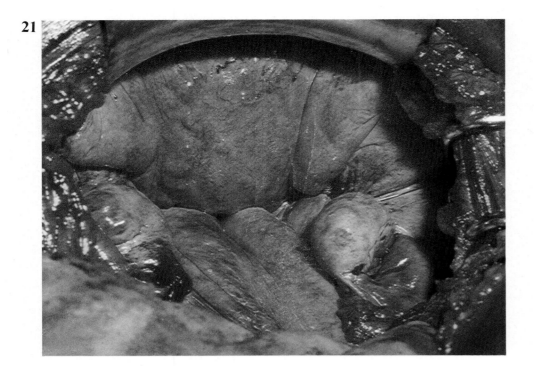

21 Closure of peritoneum
The peritoneum is shown approximated across the floor of the pelvis.

22

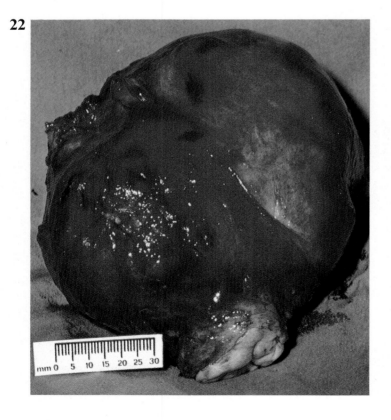

22 Specimen
The anterior view of the specimen and the position of the right round ligament shows that the fibroid arises from the lower lateral aspect of the body of the uterus and quite clear of the cervix itself.

Conditions demanding modification of basic hysterectomy technique: cervical fibroid

Fibroids on the lower anterior aspect of the uterus probably always originate in the isthmus of the uterus rather than in the cervix itself. That they are clinically referred to as cervical fibroids may not be anatomically precise, but it is appropriate because they confront the surgeon with the same dangerous problem of a wide or enlarged cervix from whatever cause.

Cervical fibroids are not usually of great size but in some respects size makes for safety, because the surgeon has to get rid of the fibroid before proceeding to hysterectomy. Smaller and medium-sized fibroids distend and broaden the supravaginal cervix and the isthmus of the uterus, so that the lateral walls come to lie against the ureter on each side. The ureter itself is fixed in the parametrial tunnel at this level and cannot be conveniently lifted upwards and laterally on the peritoneum as when more posterior in the case of the broad-ligament fibroids. Therefore, there is the danger of damage if hysterectomy is carried out in such circumstances.

One sound rule applies to all cases and that is to enucleate the fibroid. Such a procedure is easy, takes only a few moments and is almost bloodless. When enucleation is completed and the cavity of the fibroid closed by a deep haemostatic stitch, the anatomy of the region returns to normal and a seemingly difficult and dangerous prospect becomes an easy hysterectomy. The authors look on this procedure as one of the simplest and the most important lessons to be learned in gynaecological surgery; for this reason they have dealt with the problem as a specific entity. The method of enucleation of fibroids to give access and make for safety in hysterectomy is no less applicable in other parts of the uterus.

Stage 1: Separation of upper uterine supports

1A
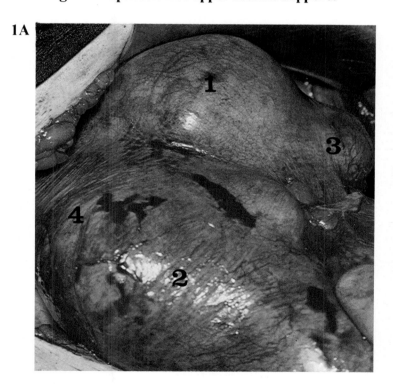

1B
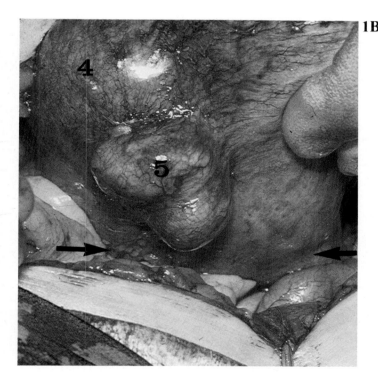

1A General view showing cervical fibroid
The cervical fibroid (1) is seen in the midline presenting between the bladder which is hidden from view behind it and the body of the uterus (2) being pulled up by the surgeon's hand. There is a smaller fibroid low on the right side (3) and a fairly large one on the left side (4).

1B General view: posterior aspect of uterus
The left-sided fibroid (4) is still visible and a further posterior fibroid (5) comes into view as the uterus is anteverted. Note the very broad lower uterus (between arrows) indicating the technical problem of the hysterectomy procedure.

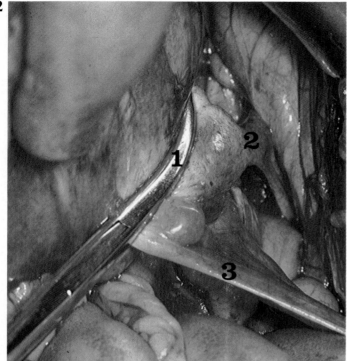

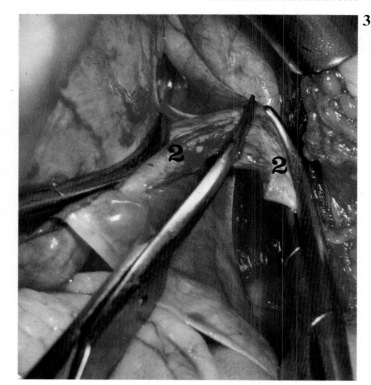

2 to 4 Dividing upper uterine attachments (right)

The right broad ligament is clamped close to the uterus (1) in Figure 2 and the thickened round ligament (2) and the fallopian tube (3) are seen. The round ligament has been clamped and is being cut (2) in Figure 3; in Figure 4 the clamped and detached broad-ligament pedicle is being ligated (4). The already ligated round ligament (2) is visible in Figure 4.

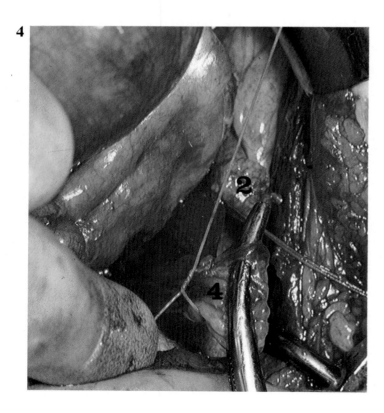

5

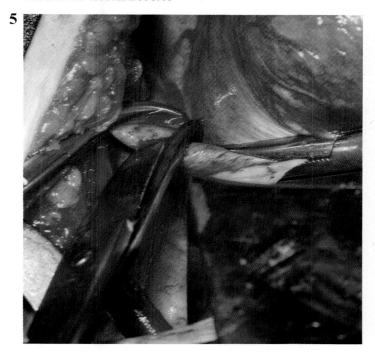

6

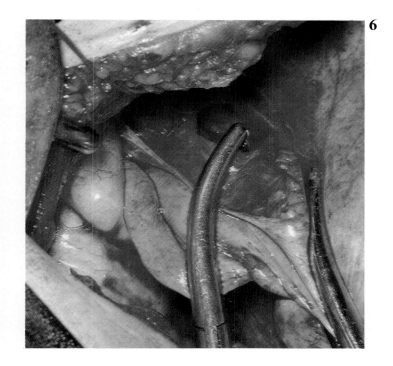

5 to 7 Dividing upper uterine attachments (left)

The left round ligament has been clamped and is being detached in Figure 5; the left broad ligament is being clamped in Figure 6 and subsequently ligated in Figure 7.

7

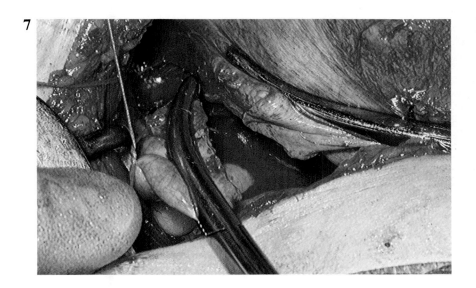

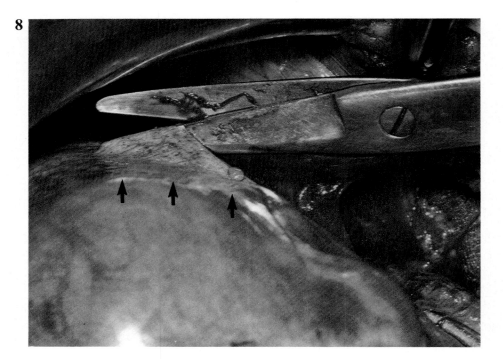

8 Opening uterovesical pouch

With the uterus retracted in a cephalad direction the loose peritoneum of the uterovesical pouch is being opened transversely just below the level of its firm attachment to the uterus (arrowed). Note that the fibroid is raising the peritoneum and obliterating the actual pouch just under the scissors.

Stage 2: Enucleation of cervical fibroid

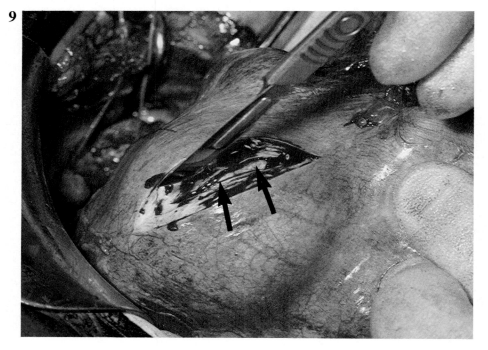

9 Incision into cervical fibroid

This figure shows the first step in excision of the fibroid and in this instance the incision is made boldly into the upper pole of the fibroid; the lower pole extends down behind the retractor towards the cervix itself. The fibroid tissue is seen (arrowed) and any bleeding from uterine muscle is minimal and is disregarded.

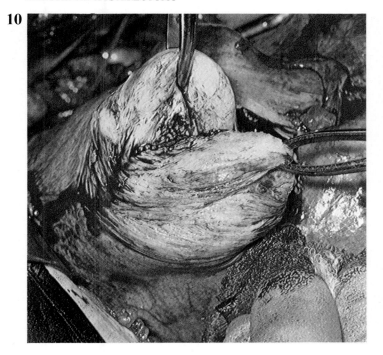

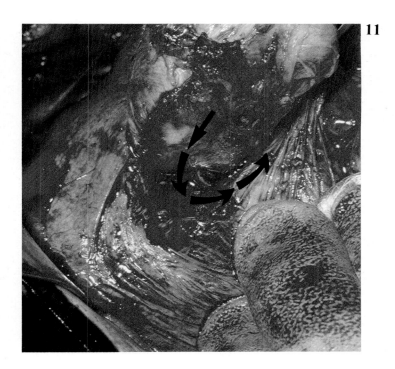

10 and 11 Enucleation of cervical fibroid

The exposed and partially bisected fibroid is grasped with Littlewood's forceps and held up firmly into the wound ready for delivery as shown in Figure 10. In Figure 11 the fibroid is partially wrenched or twisted out of its bed with the help of fingers or scissors in the direction of the arrow. While there is upward pull on the fibroid against the uterine muscle there is no bleeding.

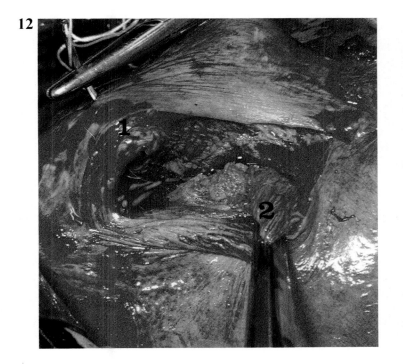

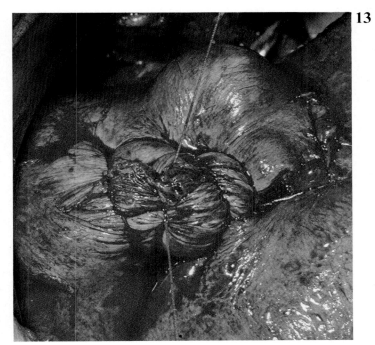

12 and 13 Closure of cavity of fibroid

The cavity left by the fibroid is closed by a deep figure-of-eight stitch which need not be placed neatly because it is temporary and its function is entirely haemostatic. In Figure 12 the first bite is being taken with the needle at (1) while the dissecting forceps (2) holds the other edge of the cavity. In Figure 13 the stitch is tied firmly, the cavity is obliterated and bleeding controlled. Note that the small fibroid on the right side is well above the level of the cervix.

14

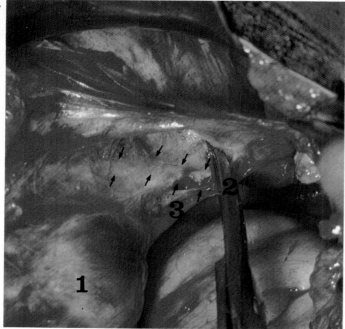

15

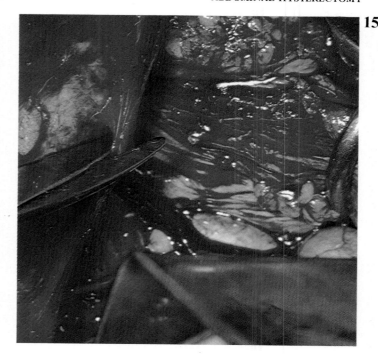

14 and 15 Definition of right ureter

In Figure 14 the small lateral fibroid (1) is held up by forceps while the scissors push the peritoneum laterally (2) and the posterior layer of the broad ligament (3) is thrown into relief.

The outline of the ureter can be just seen (arrowed). In Figure 15 the posterior layer of the broad ligament is being divided.

16

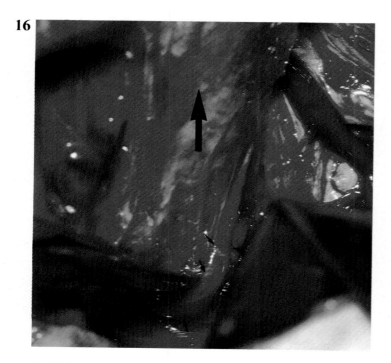

17

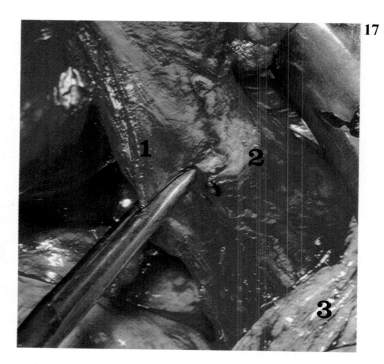

16 Right ureter displayed

The ureter is outlined lateral to the uterine vessels which are put on the stretch in the direction indicated by arrow.

17 Securing right uterine pedicle

Now that the ureter has been seen the uterine vessels (1) can be clamped off at a safe distance as seen in the illustration. The cervix and bladder are marked (2) and (3).

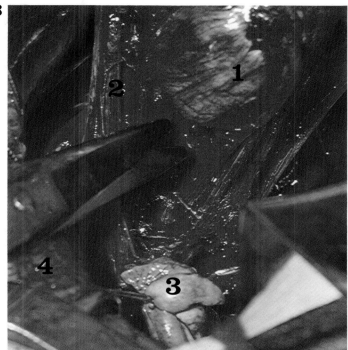

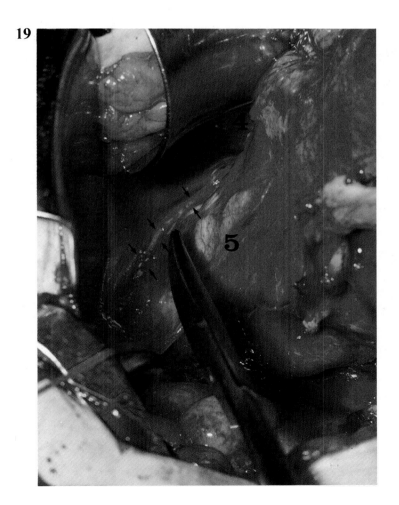

18 and 19 Visualisation of left ureter

The posterior fibroid on the left side (1) is drawn up clear of the uterine vessels (2) and these are stripped of fat and loose tissue by a downwards scissor movement as in Figure 18. The round-ligament and broad-ligament pedicles are numbered (3) and (4) respectively. In Figure 19 the ureter is seen skirting the uterus at the tip of the scissors (outlined) as it goes forwards towards the bladder (4). The cervix (5) serves as a reference point.

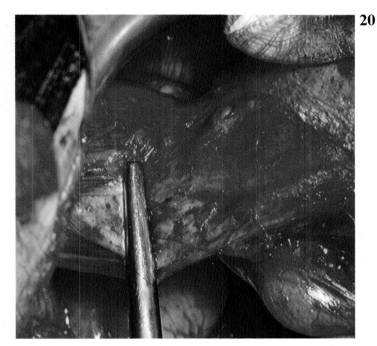

20 Securing left uterine pedicle

With knowledge of the position of the ureter the uterine vessels are safely clamped as shown. Note the posterior fibroid pulled up clear of the operation field.

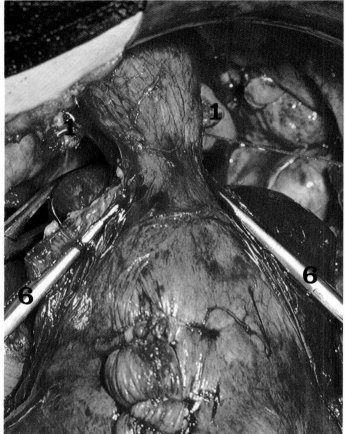

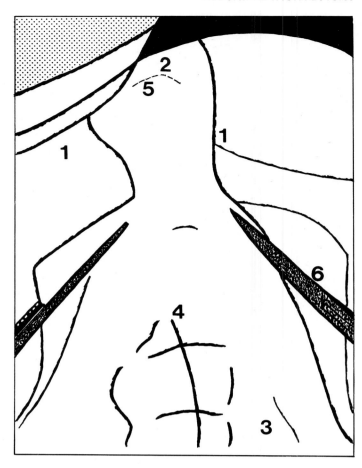

21 View from above with uterine pedicles ligated

The uterus is drawn up to put its vaginal attachment on the stretch and the ligated uterine pedicles can be seen (1). The cervix is always elongated in such cases and its lower level will be estimated between finger and thumb over the upper vagina before applying the clamping forceps to the vaginal angles.

This figure illustrates the point made in paragraph 1 of the introduction (page 83), namely that the term 'cervical fibroid' is a misnomer generally and that the fibroid in fact comes usually from the region of the isthmus of the uterus. The incision was made over the extreme upper pole of the elongated fibroid group which was then tunnelled out of the lower uterine wall. With the subsequent collapse of the distended area, it is difficult to define the lower limit of the fibroid cavity but it would extend to between the two forceps (6) preventing backflow from the uterine vessels.

Diagram numbers
1 Ligated uterine pedicle
2 Vagina
3 Uterus
4 Cavity of fibroid
5 Level of external cervical os (broken line)
6 Forceps preventing uterine backflow

Stage 4: Completion of hysterectomy

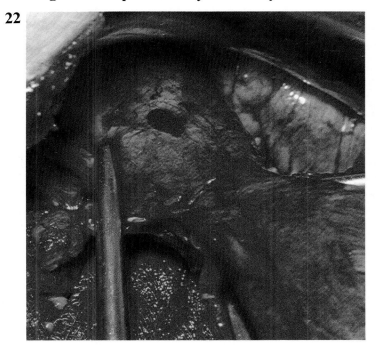

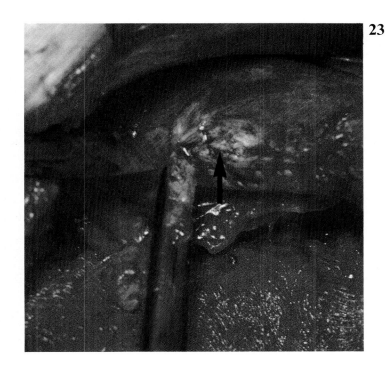

23

22 and 23 Securing left parametrium

The cervix is elongated and the cardinal ligament extends deeply alongside it, so that immediate access to the angle of the vault may not be possible. The pedicle is clamped just medial to the uterine pedicle in Figure 22 and detached from the uterus with the scalpel in Figure 23. The posterolateral fornix of the vagina has just been opened (arrowed).

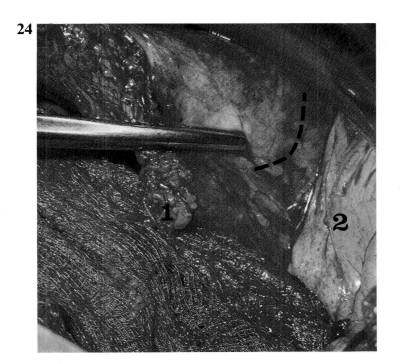

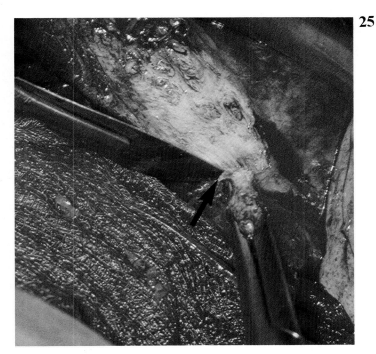

24 and 25 Securing right parametrium

The same procedure as in Figures 22 and 23 is followed on the right side and the vagina is just entered posterolaterally by the scalpel (arrowed). The ligated right uterine pedicle (1) and the bladder (2) are seen; the line of the external cervical os is marked by a broken line.

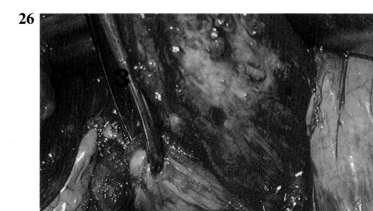

26 Posterior fornix of vagina opened

The Littlewood's forceps (1) and (2) retract the posterior edge of the vaginal vault which has now been opened, while the forceps (3) pulls the cervix posteriorly and puts the anterior and anterolateral aspects of the vagina on the stretch.

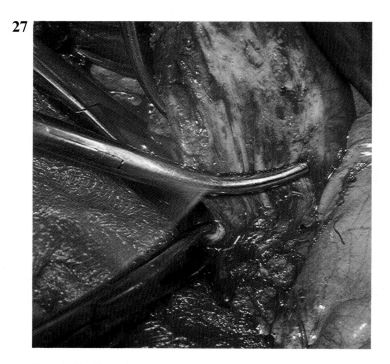

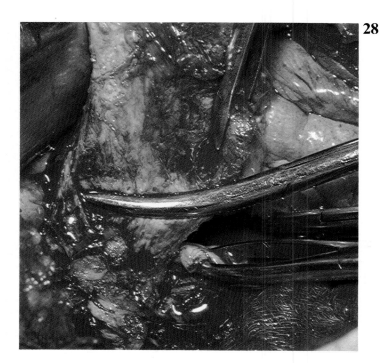

27 and 28 Clamping lateral angles of vagina

In Figure 27 the right vaginal angle and in Figure 28 the left vaginal angle are secured in forceps before detaching the uterus from the vagina.

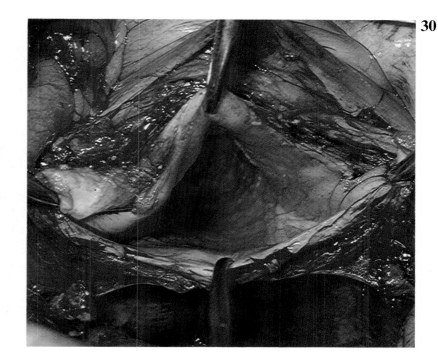

30

29 to 31 Removal of uterus and closure of vaginal vault

In Figure 29 the uterus (1) is being detached from the anterior vaginal edge (2) with scissors. In Figure 30 the open vaginal vault is seen; in Figure 31 it has been closed by mattress sutures which are still uncut.

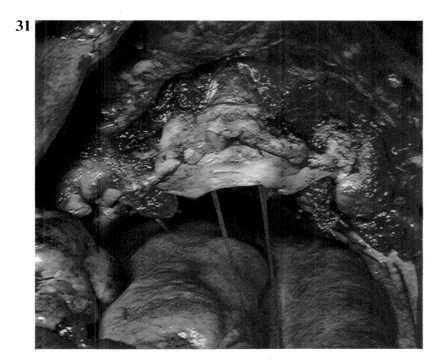

31

32

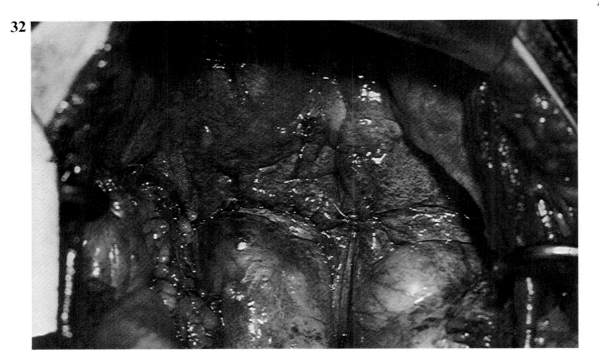

32 Closure of pelvic peritoneum

The peritoneum has been closed across the pelvic floor to cover the field of the operation; haemostasis is seen to be satisfactory.

33

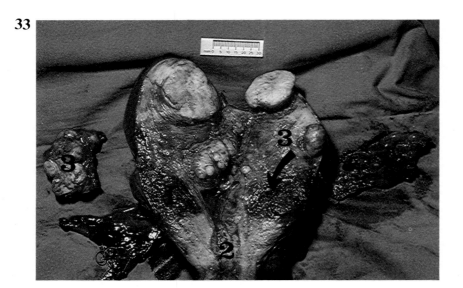

33 Specimen

The uterus contains multiple fibroids causing considerable distortion but the myomectomy done during the operation has restored the lower uterine anatomy to normal. The myomectomy incision (1) over the upper pole is seen to be well above the cervix (2). The cavity occupied by the enucleated group of fibroids (3) has not been opened fully but does not extend to the cervix.

Conditions demanding modification of basic hysterectomy technique: pelvic endometriosis

Chronic endometriosis requiring hysterectomy is a well known clinical entity. In the classic case the patient is about 40 years of age; she has a long history of dysmenorrhoea and dyspareunia, sometimes with menorrhagia. On examination there is general pelvic tenderness with an adnexal mass on one or both sides and laparoscopy may have confirmed the diagnosis. Medical therapy designed to produce a pseudo-pregnancy effect on the endometriotic lesion may have been tried and many cases are treated with the antigonadotrophin, danazol. When medical treatment has failed or the size of the lesions indicate that it will probably do so hysterectomy is the correct procedure.

In a preoperative discussion regarding ovarian involvement it is unwise to be over-sanguine about conservation. The surgeon must have a mandate to do what is thought best at operation; he may think it prudent to explain that a hormone implant or exogenous oral oestrogens will prevent meno-pausal symptoms. Recurrence of pain and dyspareunia can come from a very normal looking ovary; a further operation to remove it can leave both patient and surgeon dissatisfied with past performance.

Regarding surgical technique the textbooks give a daunting description of probable difficulties and heroic expedients which are somewhat out of date. Whether because patients demand earlier relief or because of the universal use of progestogens for contraception and pain relief, it is a welcome development that the really solid endometriotic pelvis is now rarely seen; the operation is less hazardous than that for chronic pelvic inflammatory disease. Adhesions and fibrosis occur in response to peritoneal irritation by the recurring escape of sterile blood, but are generally both light and easily separated by blunt dissection. The surface of the peritoneum only is affected and although there are obvious adhesions the process does not normally extend extraperitoneally. If the planes of cleavage are sought carefully within the peritoneal cavity and care is taken not to breach that membrane, it is possible to release the appendages from the side wall of the pelvis and the back of the broad ligament and elevate them into the wound. Chocolate cysts will always be opened in doing so, because their capsule is formed by adhesions which have to be broken down. Endometriosis in the pouch of Douglas and at the attachments of the uterosacral ligaments usually causes retroversion of the uterus with a certain amount of fixation and attachment of the rectum at the vault posteriorly. This is dealt with by holding the uterus bodily upwards and forwards, while separating the rectum by cutting the adhesions close to the uterus. This is done with the points of the curved scissors facing away from the rectum and actually cutting into the uterine wall rather than imperil the rectum; usually, however, a plain of cleavage emerges. As the rectum falls away backwards the uterosacral ligaments are encountered and are boldly cut through and detached without attempting to clamp them with forceps. Any bleeding points on the free cut ends can be sealed with diathermy if required. With that done, the uterus is released and comes up easily from the pelvic floor to allow hysterectomy to be completed.

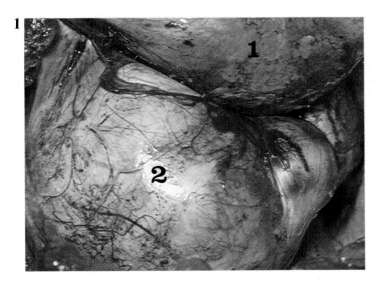 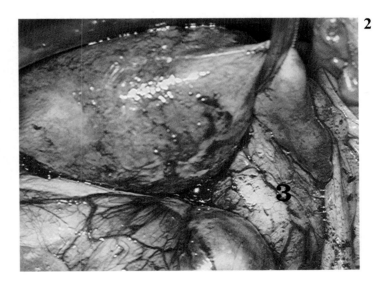

1 and 2 General view: endometriotic cysts

In Figure 1 the forceps on the broad ligament hold up the uterus (1) into the abdominal wound and an adherent left ovarian cyst (2) is seen. When the forceps on the left side is removed in Figure 2 the left-sided cyst moves laterally to show one of similar size underneath and arising from the right ovary (3).

3

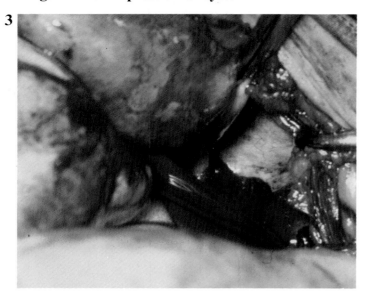

4

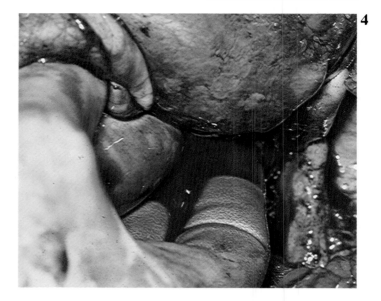

3 to 5 Draining contents from chocolate cysts

There is no question of being able to preserve the cysts intact during surgery; it is better to be rid of the contents immediately so that the anatomy is partially restored to normal. In Figure 3 elevation of the uterus by the forceps on the broad ligaments was enough to release a gush of chocolate-coloured fluid trapped between the left ovary and the posterior wall of the uterus. In Figure 4 the surgeon's forefinger is exploring under the right cyst before elevating it and the cyst contents are beginning to escape. In Figure 5 the whole pelvis is filled with fluid which is being removed with a sucker.

5

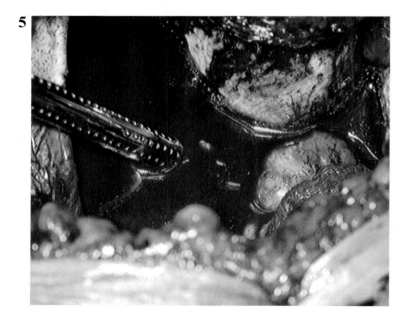

Stage 2: Elevation of appendages

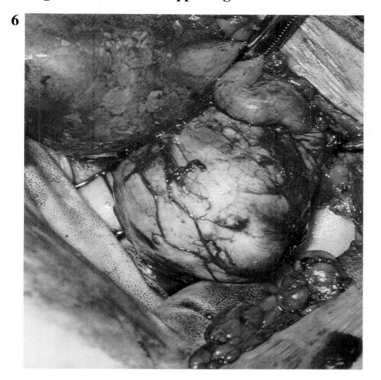

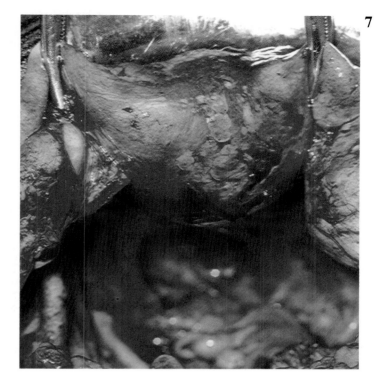

6 and 7 Elevation of appendages

The most important manoeuvre in the operation is elevation of the decompressed appendages; this is achieved by digital blunt separation of the appendages from the pelvic floor in the first instance. The appendages on each side are then raised upwards and medially towards the fundus of the uterus while separating them from the side wall of the pelvis. Adhesions are seldom strong and it is most unusual not to quickly find the plane of cleavage. As already explained the peritoneum has not been breached and is left intact after separation, although there is adherent organised blood and debris which suggests that there is a raw surface when in fact there is not. In Figure 6 the right appendages have been freed; in Figure 7 both right and left appendages have been delivered into the wound. The pelvic floor looks surprisingly healthy.

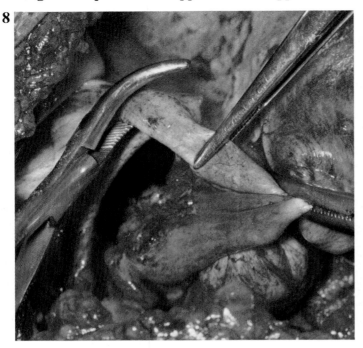

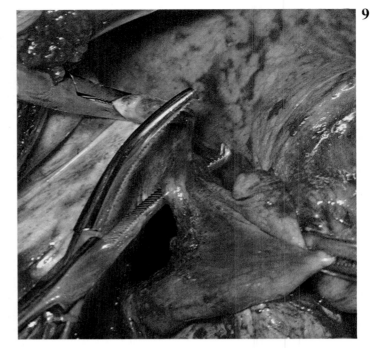

8 to 11 Separation of upper uterine attachments

Hysterectomy can now proceed. In Figure 8 the left round ligament is being clamped; in Figure 9 the left ovarian pedicle is being secured. In Figure 10 the right round ligament and in Figure 11 the right ovarian pedicle is being clamped.

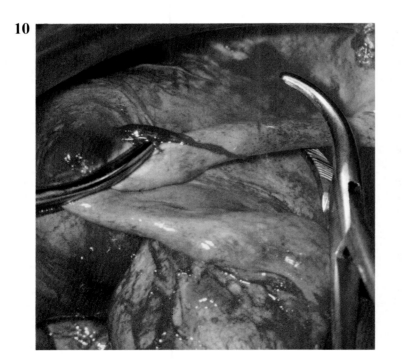

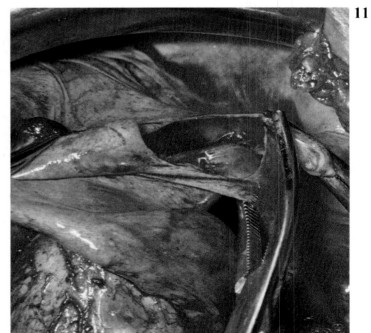

12

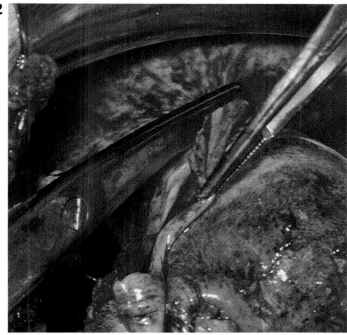

12 to 14 Securing uterine pedicles

In Figure 12 the uterovesical pouch is being opened. In Figure 13 the uterine vessels on the left are being clamped; in Figure 14 the right uterine pedicle is being detached from the uterus. The uterine vessels are seen clearly (1) in the clamped pedicle, while the round ligament is numbered (2) and the ovarian pedicle (3).

13

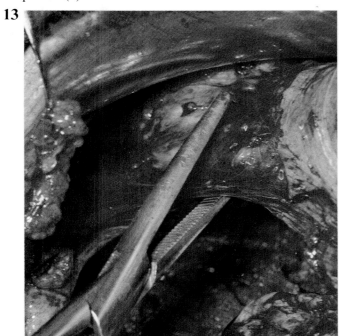

14

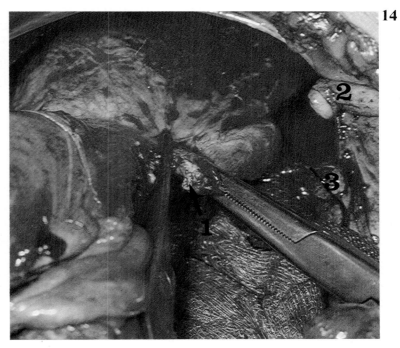

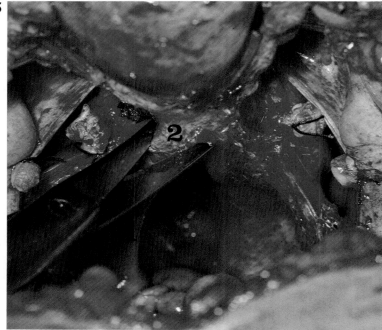

15 to 17 Separation of uterus posteriorly

It is to be expected that the endometriotic process will involve the uterine attachments of the uterosacral ligaments and probably the anterior surface of the rectum at that level. Figure 15 shows the left uterosacral ligament (1) being divided sufficiently far from the uterus to be clear of the endometriotic tissue (2). The same procedure is carried out on the other side in Figure 16 with the corresponding tissues numbered (3) and (4). In Figure 17 the rectum (5) has been detached from the uterus clear of the endometriotic tissue on the uterus (6). The uterine pedicles (7) are also seen.

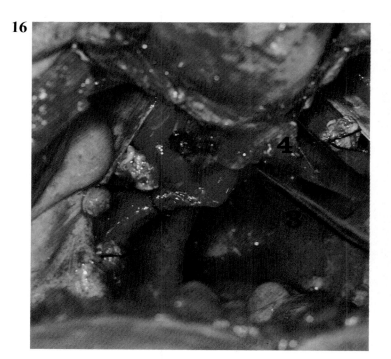

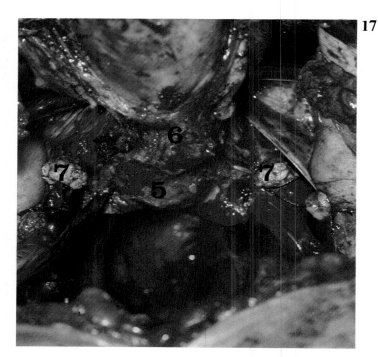

18

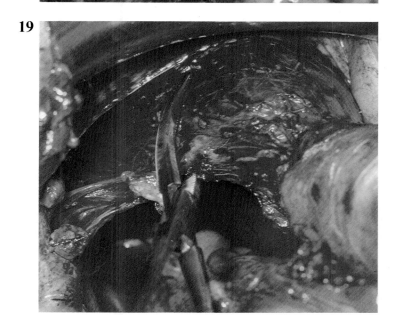

18 Separation of bladder from uterus
The bladder is separated off the front of the cervix in the usual fashion. Endometriosis does not usually cause problems of adhesion in this area. The uterine vessels are shown clearly in the pedicle (arrowed).

19

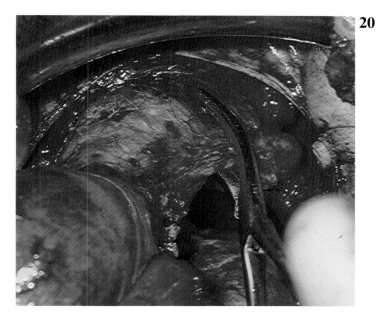

20

21

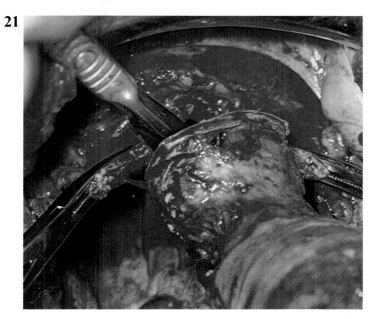

19 to 21 Securing vaginal angles and removing uterus
The left vaginal angle is being clamped in Figure 19, the right in Figure 20; the uterus is being detached from the vagina with the scalpel in Figure 21. Note that the uterus is now coming up into the wound easily and there is no problem of fixation.

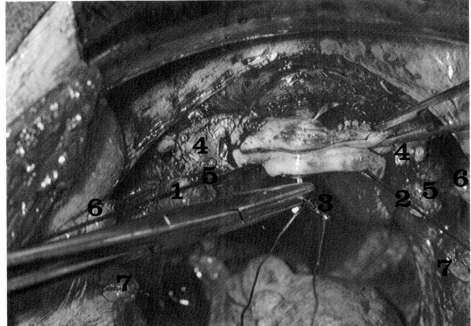

22 Closure of vaginal vault

The two angles of the vault have been closed and the inner mattress sutures are being used as holders, (1) and (2). The first stage of a central mattress suture is being placed (3).

Numbers indicate the various pedicles thus: (4) vaginal angle, (5) uterine vessels, (6) round ligaments and (7) ovarian pedicles.

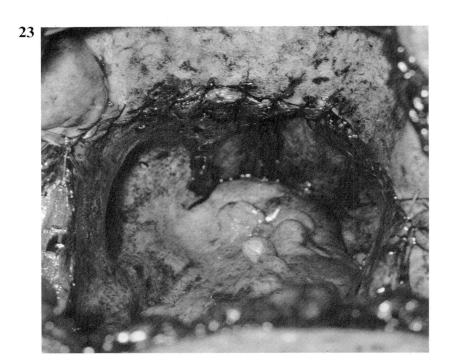

23 Closure of pelvic peritoneum

The peritoneum has come together neatly to cover the pelvic floor and side walls. It is surprising how clean the pelvis appears at the end of this type of operation.

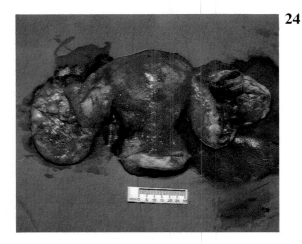

24 Specimen

The ruptured endometriotic cysts and the lower posterior uterine involvement gives the typical appearance of advanced pelvic endometriosis. A degree of adenomyosis is almost invariable in such cases.

Conditions demanding modification of basic hysterectomy technique: chronic pelvic inflammatory disease

The most likely cause of hazardous pelvic surgery or hysterectomy is previous pelvic inflammatory disease. Such infections have several aetiologies and the severity and amount of damage done varies enormously. However, all tend to produce unacceptable symptoms and accompanying physical signs which lead to hysterectomy.

A common feature of such cases is that in addition to the uterus and appendages the pelvic viscera and the pelvic peritoneum are involved and there is widespread adhesion and fibrosis. The bladder is not usually involved even in severe cases because the uterus lies between it and the source of infection.

In the text, illustrations from a mild, a moderate and a severe case are shown in turn. The approach is generally similar in all; the severity of the condition dictates the extent of the dissection required. It need not be emphasised that these can be very difficult operations; it is absolutely essential to proceed slowly and cautiously with constant reference to the vascular and particularly the ureteric anatomy.

Mild case of pelvic inflammatory disease

In less severe cases the appendages are inflamed, enlarged and damaged but relatively easy to mobilise and pelvic clearance is not difficult. The bowel will be adherent to some extent but should not cause undue difficulty. The group may for convenience be classified as 'mild' and treatment is relatively straightforward. A note of caution should perhaps be added regarding closure of the pelvic peritoneum in such cases. It is very easy to catch or distort the ureter in making a neat pelvic covering; this danger is seen in the case described.

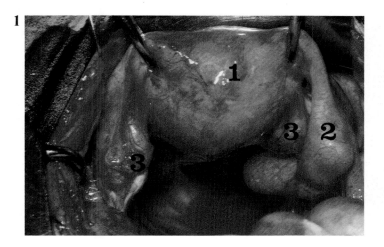

1 General view of chronic pelvic sepsis (posterior)
The uterus (1) is elevated from the pelvic floor with tissue forceps to show a right hydrosalpinx (2) and the ovaries (3) covered with adhesions which extend across the back of the uterus down to the pouch of Douglas.

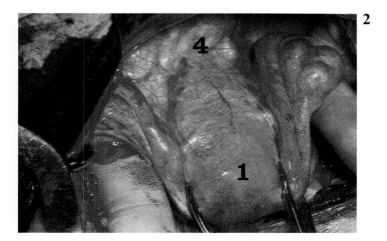

2 General view of chronic pelvic sepsis (anterior)
From this view it is seen that the bladder (4) and the anterior aspect of the uterus (1) are not involved. The elevated appendages on each side show the chronic infection from this aspect.

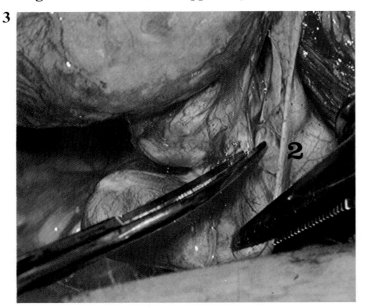

3 and 4 Mobilisation of right hydrosalpinx

As already mentioned, the primary aim is to elevate the affected appendages from the pelvis and in Figure 3 the hydrosalpinx (2) is being freed from adhesions medially; in Figure 4 it is pulled forward and laterally in the direction of the arrow while the scissors separate it from the pelvic floor and side wall of the pelvis. The ureter (3) comes into view as its covering peritoneum is detached with the adherent appendages, but it is not endangered by the subsequent procedure.

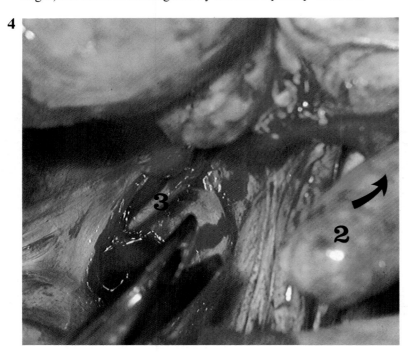

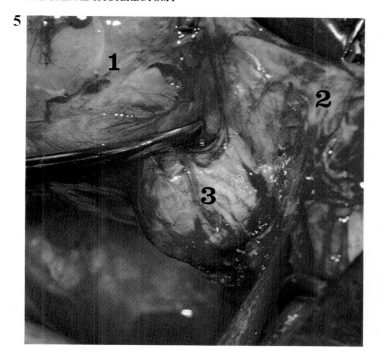

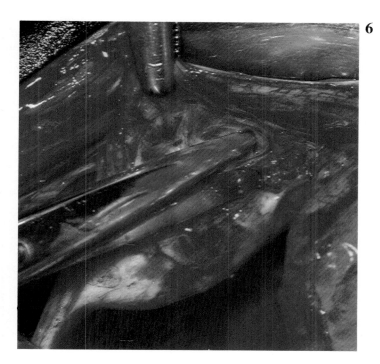

5 Mobilisation of right ovary

With the hydrosalpinx (2) elevated the adhesions between the uterus (1) and the ovary (3) are divided with scissors.

6 Mobilisation of left tube and ovary

A similar procedure is carried out on the less affected left side.

Stage 2: Separation of upper uterine supports and vessels

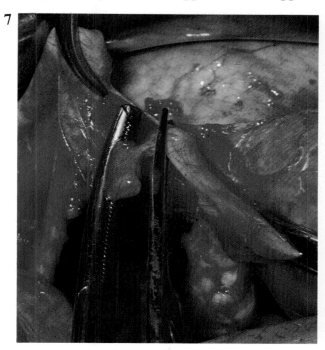

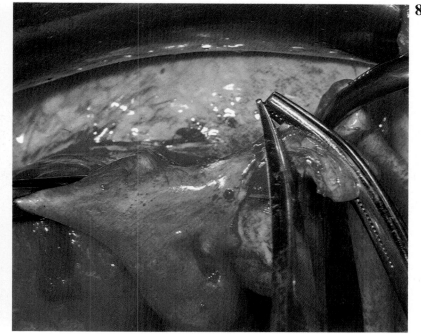

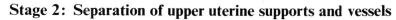

7 and 8 Division of upper uterine attachments

Hysterectomy proceeds with detachment of round ligaments and ovarian pedicles; Figure 7 shows the ovarian pedicle being divided on the left side; Figure 8 shows the same step on the right.

9

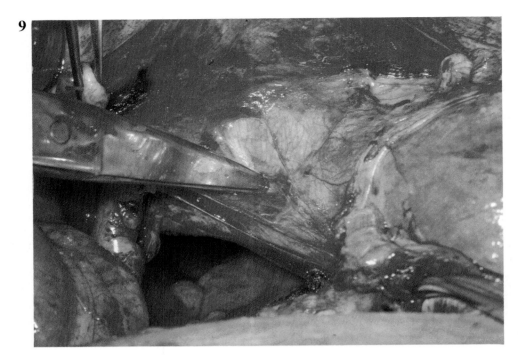

9 Definition of left uterine vessels

The uterus comes up freely into the wound and there is no apparent danger to the ureters although the uterine pedicles are nonetheless carefully defined.

10

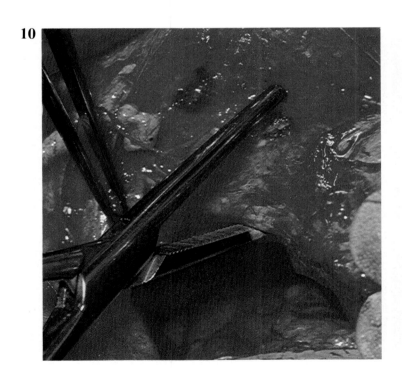

11

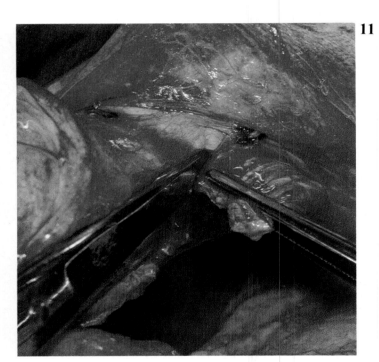

10 and 11 Securing uterine pedicles

The left uterine vessels are clamped in Figure 10 and the pedicle is being detached on the right side in Figure 11. The point of the forceps in the latter case is being freed close to the uterus so that the pedicle can be levered down on the forceps to give a good length of pedicle for ligation.

Stage 3: Separation and ligation of lower uterine supports

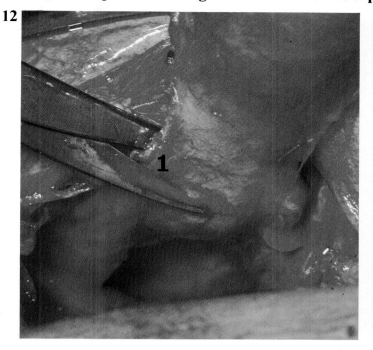

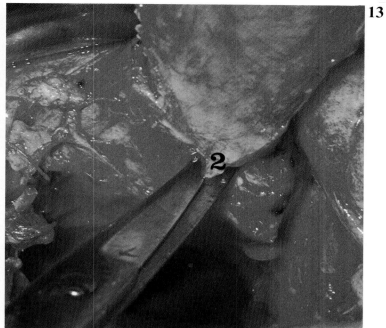

12 to 14 Detaching uterus posteriorly

The left uterosacral ligament (1) is cut with scissors in Figure 12 and the same is done on the right (2) in Figure 13. In Figure 14 the peritoneum has been stripped downwards and backwards off the uterus and it can be seen that the rectum (3)

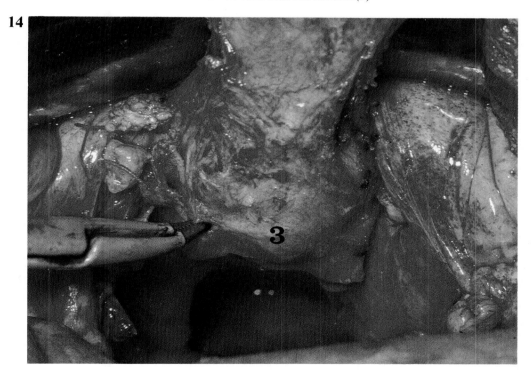

underlies the edge at no great distance. The uterosacral ligaments have not been clamped before separation in this case; the reader will notice that the authors may omit this step occasionally. There are sometimes advantages in having the structures displayed openly with an absence of attached forceps and ligatures, especially if the vault does not need reinforcement. Bleeding is not a problem; diathermy seals off any small arteries in the cut ligament as shown in Figure 14.

15

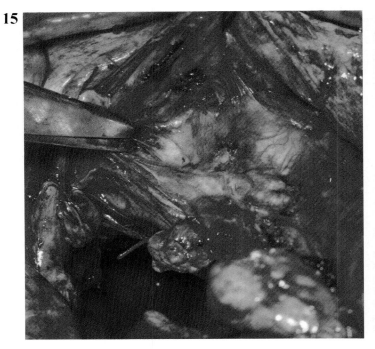

16

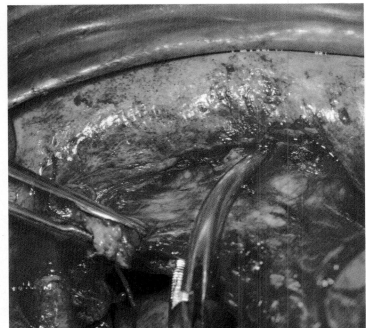

15 and 16 Further steps in hysterectomy (1)
The bladder is separated off the cervix in Figure 15 and the left
vaginal angle is clamped in Figure 16.

17

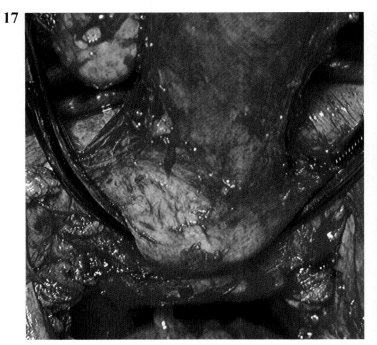

18

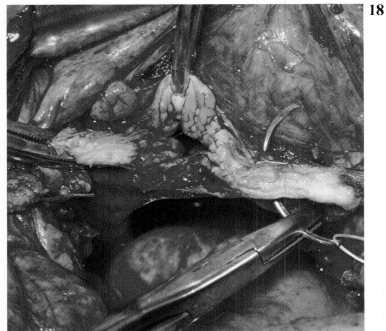

17 and 18 Further steps in hysterectomy (2)
A posterior view shows the angles secured in Figure 17 and in
Figure 18 the uterus has been removed and the right angle of
the vault is being closed.

Stage 4: Peritoneal closure

19

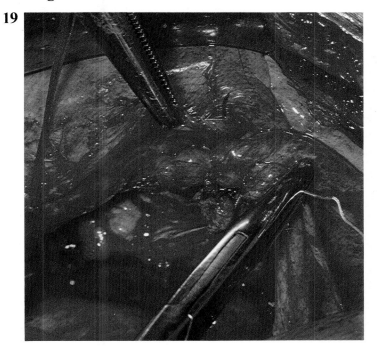

20

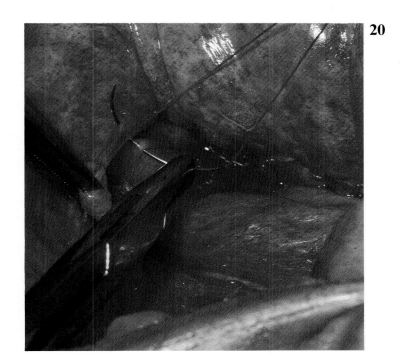

19 and 20 Closure of pelvic peritoneum
Figure 19 shows the round ligament and ovarian pedicle being buried by a half purse-string suture before carrying the stitch across the pelvic floor. There is a deficiency of normal healthy peritoneum because of the inflammatory process; in Figure 20 the visceral peritoneum on the anterior aspect of the rectum is used as a substitute.

21

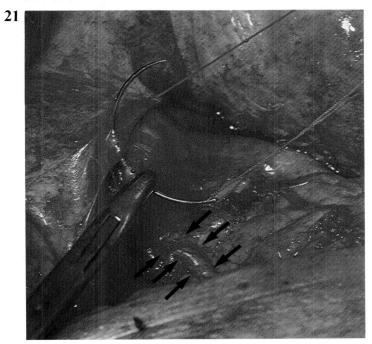

22

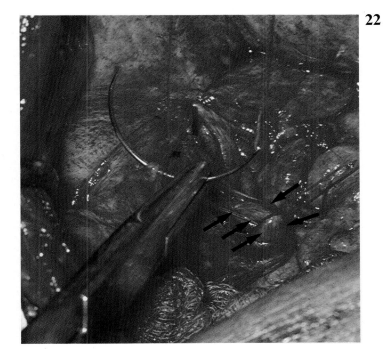

21 and 22 Attention to ureter in peritoneal closure
Although the ureter did not obtrude on the operation it comes into view at this stage and could be caught up in the peritoneal stitch especially where there is a dearth of peritoneum. The best way of avoiding such a danger is always to pick up the edge of the peritoneal leaf only and not try to infold it. The ureter is outlined in the two photographs.

Moderate case of pelvic inflammatory disease

Where there is firm adhesion of the appendages to the floor of the pelvis, fibrosis distorts and alters the anatomy of the ureters as they traverse the pelvis. Great care is essential in mobilising the structures in such cases, but once the adherent appendages have been elevated from the pelvic floor and it is known where the ureters lie hysterectomy becomes relatively straightforward. This group can be classified as 'moderately severe'. The essential manoeuvre in treatment is first to free and raise the bowel from the pelvis in a cephalad direction and gradually release the adherent appendages from the pouch of Douglas and pelvic side walls, so that they eventually come up to their correct anatomical position. Care is taken to avoid opening the bowel but that may not be possible; in such circumstances it is closed forthwith as will be described in the text. Release of the appendages must be gentle and usually entails a certain amount of sharp dissection where they are adherent to the pelvic floor and to the posterior aspect of the uterus. A continual search is made for a plane of separation which is then developed to free the structure from the pelvic peritoneum. If one keeps within the peritoneal cavity then the ureter will be safe, but it is more than likely that the integrity of the peritoneum will at some point have been violated. The safest procedure when running into potential trouble is to definitively find the ureter on each side and perhaps underrun it with a tape as a marker until dissection is complete.

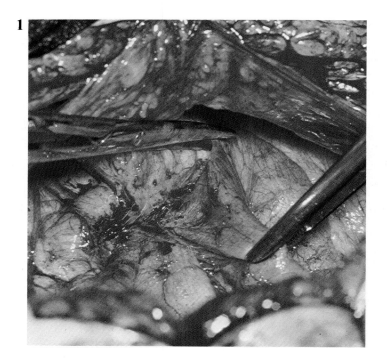

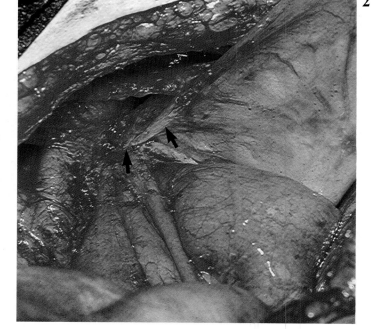

1 and 2 General view of chronic pelvic sepsis
The uterus and appendages are buried under a covering of small intestine in this case but omentum and large intestine are also usually present. A loop of bowel is held in dissecting forceps while fine adhesions are divided with fine scissors in Figure 1. In Figure 2 a closer view with the bowel elevated shows where a plane of cleavage will be sought (arrowed).

Stage 1: Mobilisation of appendages

3

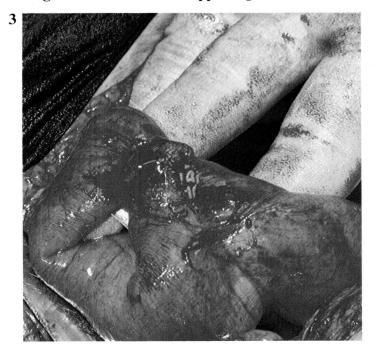

4

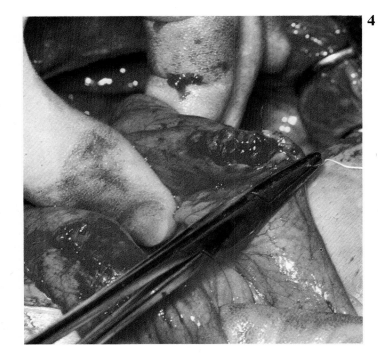

3 to 5 Mobilisation and repair of injured small intestine

Figure 3 shows matted adhesion of several coils of small intestine which require further separation. In Figure 4 unavoidable damage to the bowel wall is being repaired. Even if the mucosa has not been opened as in this case the intestine should be closed in two layers; this should be done at right angles to the line of the instestine so that there is no question of subsequent narrowing of the lumen. PGA No. 00 suture is used to make a through-and-through closure of all coats and taking up minimal mucosa. In Figure 5 a Lembert continuous inverting suture is used to complete the closure. The bowel is examined carefully; where there is any damage to the serosal coat a similar Lembert suture is inserted.

5

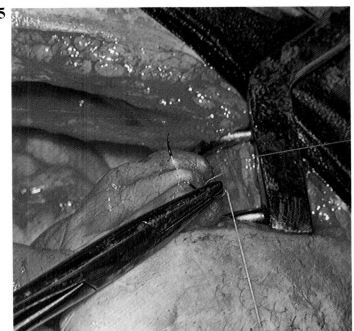

6

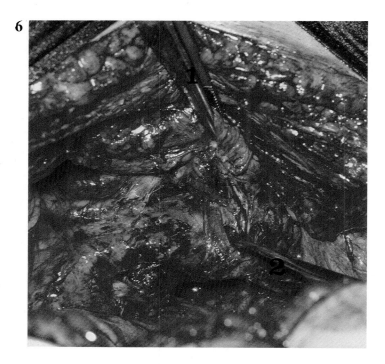

6 General view following separation of intestine
The thickened anterior peritoneum is held in dissecting
forceps (1) while the fundus of the uterus is drawn back by
tissue forceps (2) to show the degree of adhesion.

7

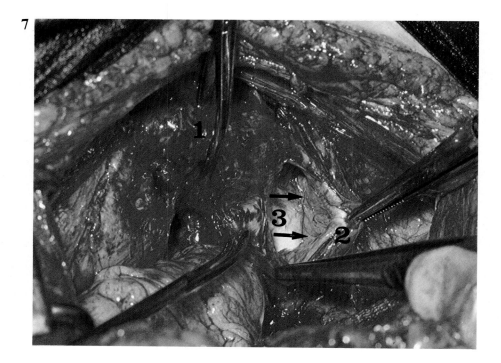

7 Mobilisation of right appendages (1)
As in the previous case the uterus (1) is held medially and
upwards while the right tube (2) is separated laterally off the
surface of the right ovary (3) by sharp dissection. A plane of
separation is becoming obvious where arrowed.

8

9

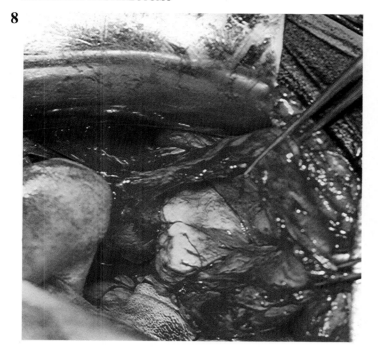

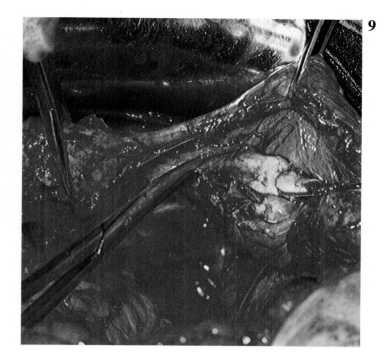

8 and 9 Mobilisation of right appendages (2)

The process of mobilisation is effected by a combination of sharp and blunt dissection while at the same time lifting up the structures by the attached forceps.

10

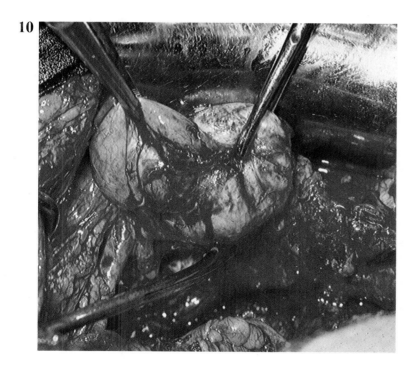

10 Mobilisation of left appendages

The same procedure is carried out on the left side and the fine scissors are dividing para-ovarian adhesions.

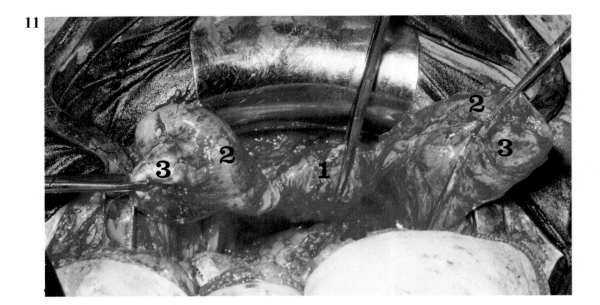

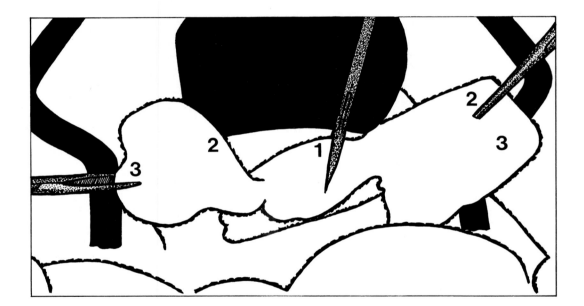

11 Uterus and appendages mobilised

With the appendages freed and elevated into the wound the body of the uterus itself can be pulled up although there is usually considerable fixation at the vaginal vault posteriorly; this will have to be dealt with later. For the moment hysterectomy can proceed. The structures are labelled thus: ureters (1); tubes (2); ovaries (3).

Stage 2: Separation of upper uterine supports

12

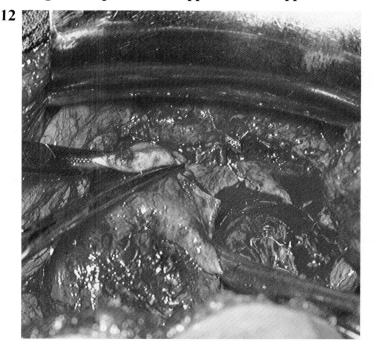

13

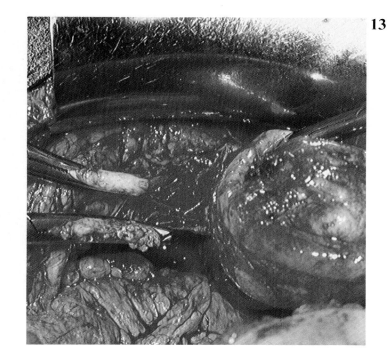

12 to 15 Division of upper uterine attachments

The upper uterine attachments are secured and divided in turn. In Figure 12 the left round ligament is being cut, in Figure 13 both it and the ovarian pedicle are held in forceps; in Figure 14 the right round ligament pedicle and in Figure 15 the right ovarian pedicle are being clamped.

14

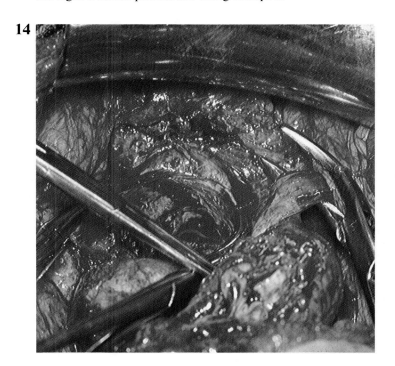

15

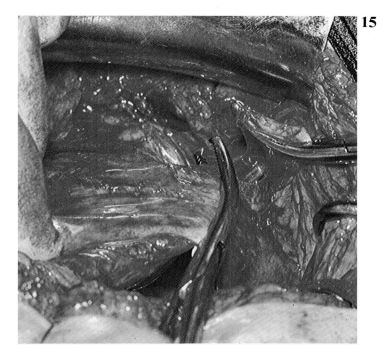

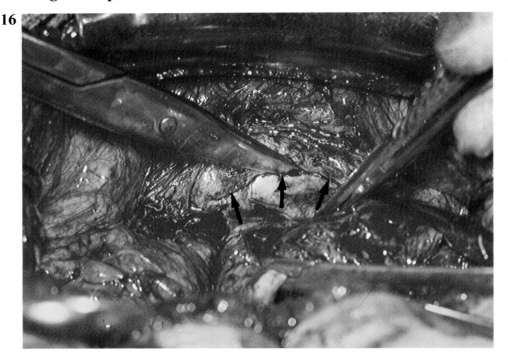

16 Separation of bladder from cervix

Despite the degree of adhesion around and posterior to the uterus the bladder is only superficially involved; separation from the uterus in the uterovesical pouch is straightforward. A good plane of separation is developing (arrowed).

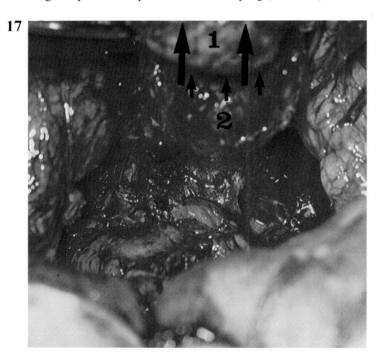

17 Separation of rectum from uterus posteriorly

The photograph shows fibrosis and adhesion between the posterior wall of the uterus (1) and the anterior wall of the rectum (2); it is essential to keep close to the uterus in separating them. The initial sharp dissection should be done against the uterus or upper cervix and even cutting into these structures if in doubt. A plane of separation can be encouraged to appear by pulling up the uterus quite firmly in the direction of the arrows and the bowel in due course falls away posteriorly. The uterosacral attachments form part of this fibrotic attachment and are recognised as firm lateral areas which are detached from the uterus with scissors. No attempt is made to definitively clamp these as they are ill-defined, of rubber-like consistency and avascular in any case. The structures of relevance are numbered thus: uterus (1), rectum (2), and the line of separation between uterus and rectum is arrowed.

18

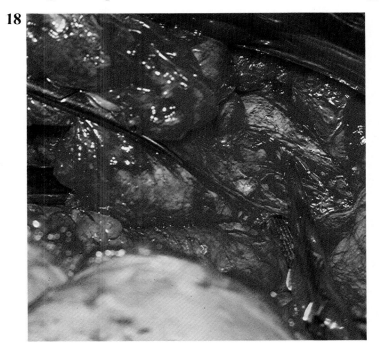

19

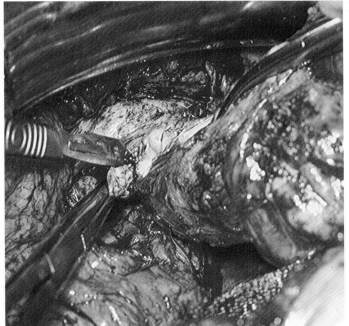

18 Securing right uterine pedicle

With the uterus and cervix freed at the vault posteriorly, the uterus is pulled up into the wound and the right uterine pedicle is carefully defined. A uterine clamp is then safely applied under direct vision.

19 Dividing left uterine pedicle

The left uterine vessels have been similarly secured and the pedicle is cut distal to the forceps with a scalpel. The separation is usually shown being done with scissors but as a result of general fibrosis in a case of this type it was found necessary to use a scalpel. The surgeon is working close to the uterus here; it is not possible to get a good cuff of tissue with the scissors.

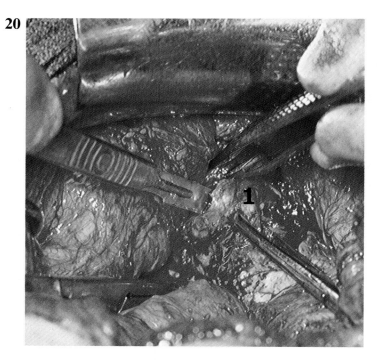

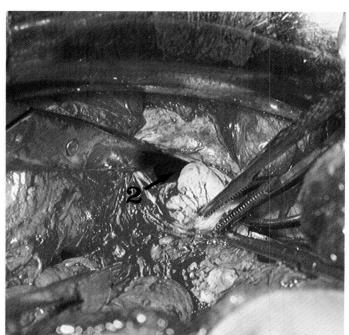

20 to 23 Removal of uterus

Because of the general fibrosis and contraction around the vault of the vagina in such cases it is unwise to insist on definitively applying forceps to the vaginal angles as one would normally do in hysterectomy. The lower renal tract has been avoided carefully thus far but the ureters are obviously at

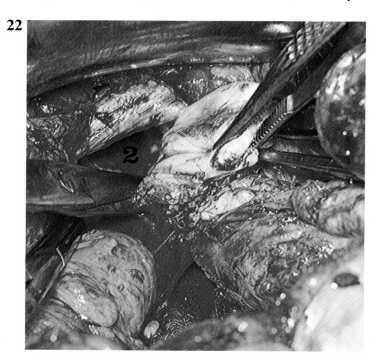

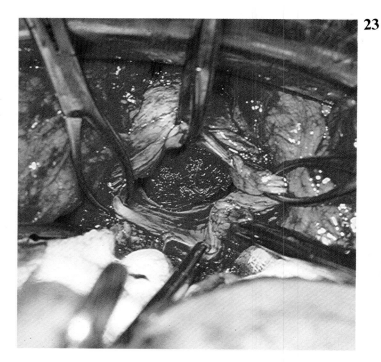

no great distance from the vault; the distortion of applying heavy forceps could bring them into danger. There is little likelihood of bleeding with the amount of fibrosis present and the method illustrated here is the safest and most satisfactory.

In Figure 20 the scalpel opens the anterior vaginal wall below the level of the cervix (1); in Figures 21 and 22 the vagina (2) is cut round with the scissors to detach the uterus and demonstrate the vaginal vault which is held open with a swab (Figure 23).

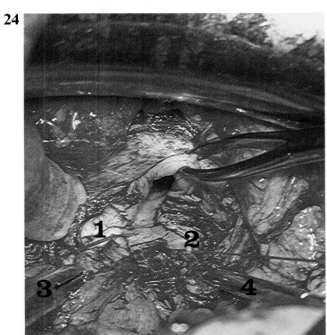

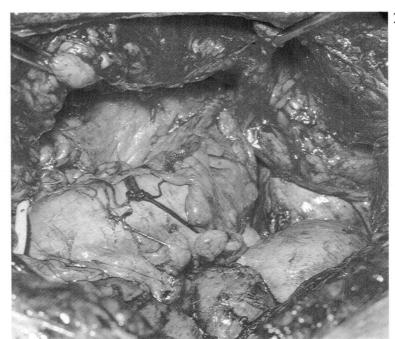

24 and 25 Completion of hysterectomy

In Figure 24 the vault of the vagina is being closed by transversely placed mattress sutures (1) and (2). The two uterine clamps (3) and (4) are still in position. In Figure 25 the closed pelvic peritoneum is shown. Note that in this case also the peritoneum on the large bowel has been brought forward to help cover the pelvic floor defect.

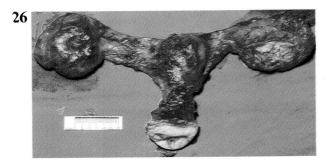

26 Specimen

The structures are all fibrotic and thickened. They are typical of long-standing chronic pelvic inflammatory disease.

Severe case of pelvic inflammatory disease

Severe cases are represented in extreme form by the frozen pelvis, an apt name for a condition where the uterus and appendages are firmly adherent to each other and to the pelvic peritoneum over the whole floor of the pelvis. These structures are hidden completely from view by a top layer of adherent small bowel, large bowel and omentum which is plastered on to them and to the bladder and is adherent to both pelvic side walls. At first sight there seems no prospect of ever unravelling such a tangle. With careful and painstaking dissection the problem can be overcome; the general principles are the same as those used for lesser degrees of pelvic sepsis.

The 'roof' of omentum and adherent bowel is separated from the pelvic brim laterally and anteriorly and folded back into the abdominal cavity where it is retained by a large moist swab. The appendages are then defined, detached and raised gently from the pelvic floor. During this stage of dissection the ureters are sought actively on each side and their position noted. Concurrently with or immediately after the freeing of the appendages the ureters are followed forward towards the parametrium and the ureteric tunnels there. Hysterectomy can now proceed. Once the base of the broad ligament has been reached the ureters are redefined and dissected out as in a Wertheim's hysterectomy. The uterine vessels and the roof of the tunnel are divided on each side and the ureters exposed in their full length. They are subsequently displaced laterally on the floor of the ureteric tunnel as far as necessary to allow safe and adequate access to the lower uterus and cervix. The bladder has meantime been separated off the front of the uterus and the hysterectomy proceeds along normal lines. It is wise to drain the pelvis in such cases, usually by means of Redivac-type drains.

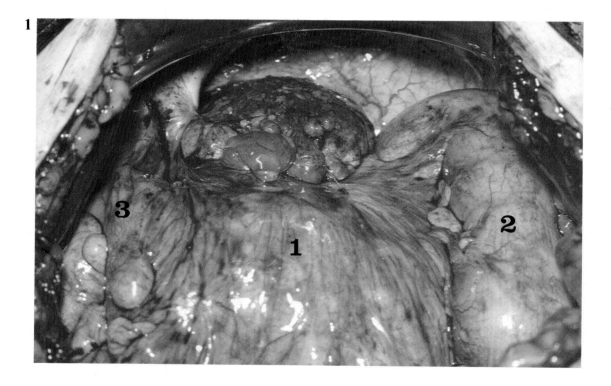

1 General view on opening abdomen
The omentum (1), small intestine (2) and large intestine (3) are all represented in the adherent structure or 'roof' which covers the chronically infected pelvis.

2

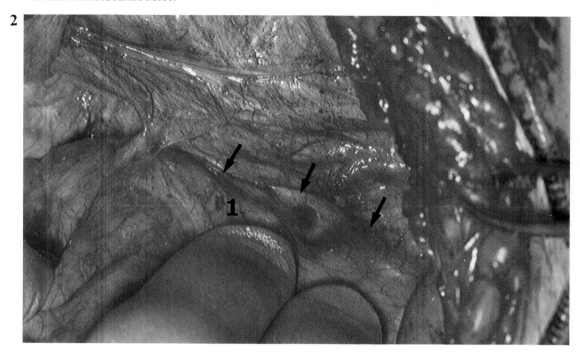

2 Appearances at right pelvic brim

The small intestine (1) is retracted medially with the fingers to show its attachment to the side of the pelvis along a line which is arrowed. A plane of separation appears likely to emerge if sought in that area.

3

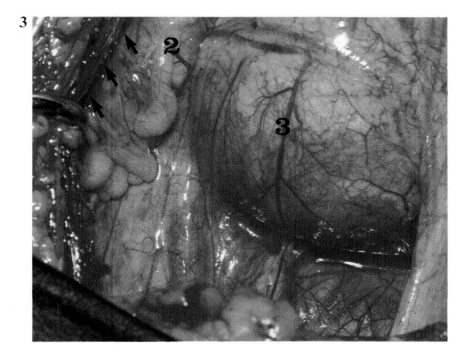

3 Appearances at left pelvic brim

The large instestine (2) covers a cystic mass in the left appendages (3) and is firmly adherent to the side of the pelvis along the line which is arrowed. Again there is the prospect of a plane of separation in that area.

4

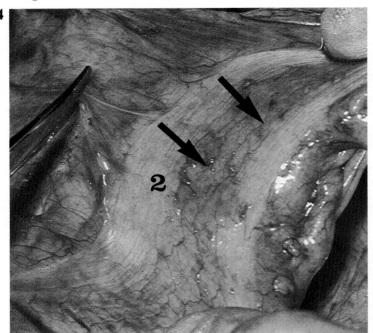

5

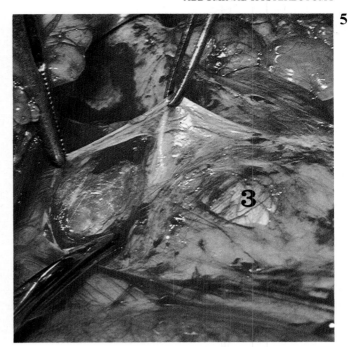

4 and 5 Mobilisation of large intestine

Because the large bowel (2) is largely central it is first freed with scissors in the plane indicated by the arrows in Figure 3 and drawn back in a cephalad direction as arrowed in Figure 4. This uncovers the cystic swelling (3) beneath and separation continues in Figure 5.

6

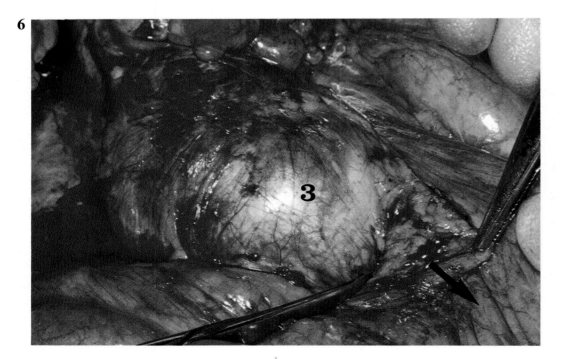

6 Exposure of cystic appendages (left)

The large bowel is further separated back to show a thin walled inflammatory type of ovarian cyst (3) attached to the back of the uterus.

7

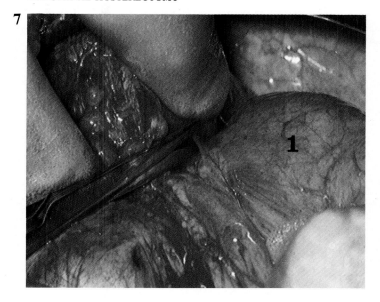

8

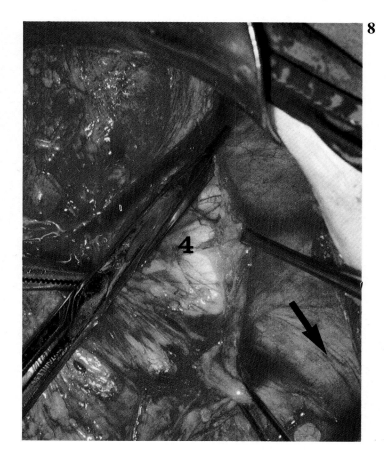

9

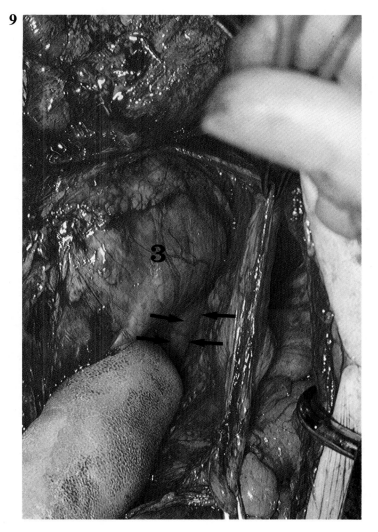

7 to 9 Mobilisation of small intestine

Transferring attention to the right side of the pelvic brim the small intestine (1) is being released anteromedially in Figure 7, swept laterally and cephalad in Figure 8 to reveal the right ovary (4); in Figure 9 it is apparent that the thin-walled cyst (3) already mentioned extends across as far as the right appendages. The ureter is seen clearly on the outer aspect of the ovarian cyst (outlined).

Stage 2: Definition of ureter

10

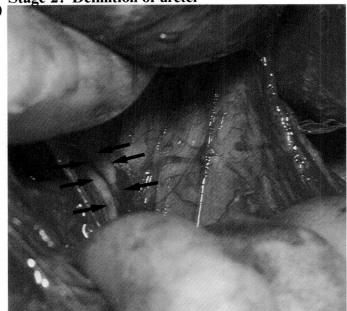

11

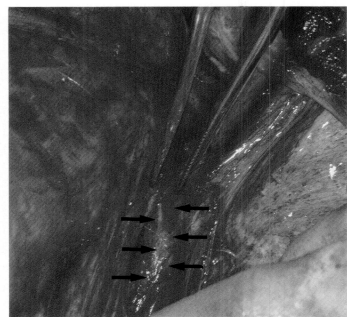

10 to 12 Exposure of right ureter

In Figure 10 the right appendages are lifted upwards and laterally to show the right ureter in the first part of its pelvic course (outlined). The structure is further defined in Figure 11 and in Figure 12 it has been underrun and elevated with a broad cotton tape (1).

12

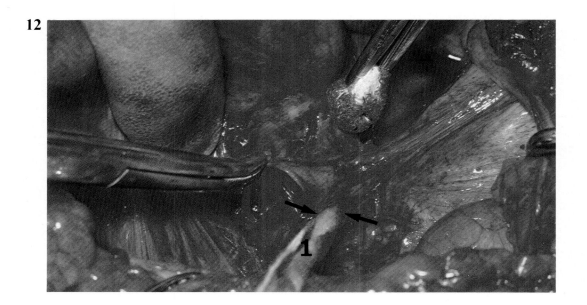

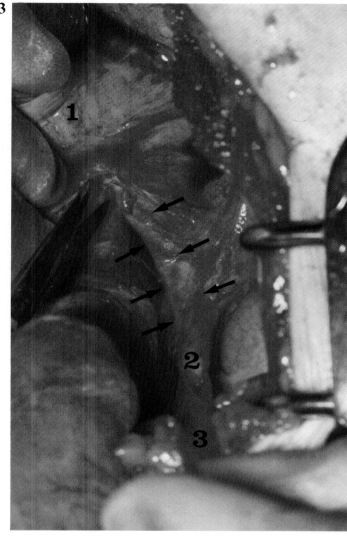

13 Separation of ureter from right appendages

The appendages (1) are held medially by the surgeon's left hand while the ureter (outlined) is freed from their lateral aspect with scissors so that it can be displaced clear of the operative area. The relevant structures are: (1) left appendages, (2) ureter, (3) tape under ureter.

14

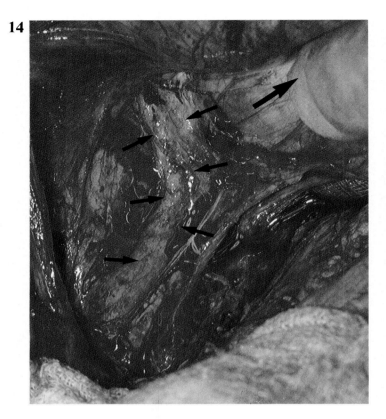

15

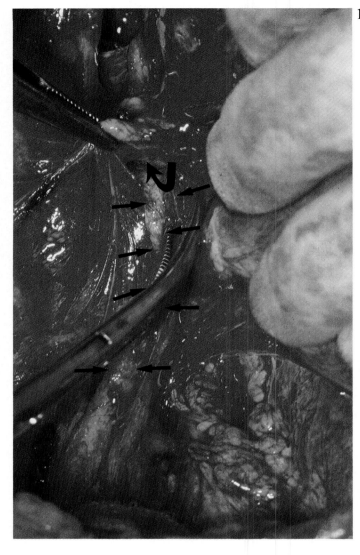

16

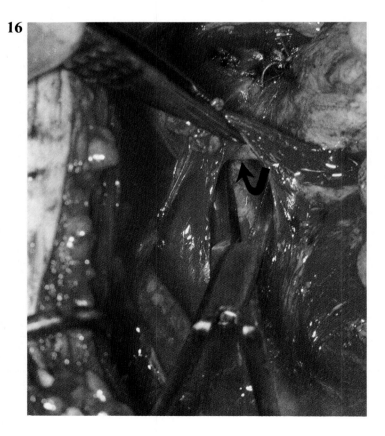

14 to 16 Exposure of left ureter

As the cystic appendages on the left side are elevated in Figure 14 (arrowed) the parietal peritoneum is torn or non-existant and the outline of the left ureter is seen clearly (outlined). The ureter is not disturbed from its mesentery or bed but is defined in this first part of its pelvic course as shown in Figure 15 and as far as its entry into the parametrial or ureteric tunnel (curved arrow). Figure 16 shows the forceps opened to display the entry of the ureter into its tunnel (curved arrow).

17

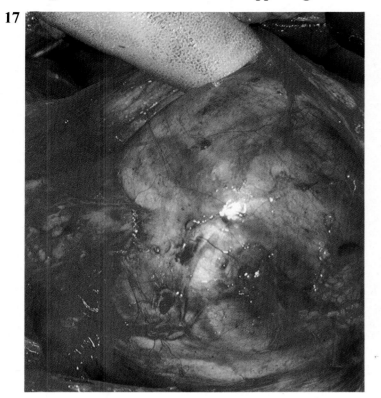

18

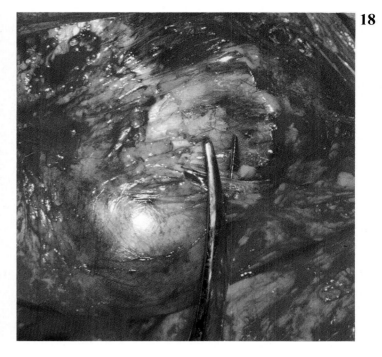

17 to 19 Mobilisation of cyst of appendages

Various stages in the mobilisation and elevation of the cystic mass are shown. In Figure 17 it is separated from the right lateral wall of the pelvis with the finger. In Figure 18 the remaining intestinal adhesions are divided with the scissors, and in Figure 19 the cyst (3) is delivered into the wound intact and attached to the posterior wall of the uterus (1) towards the left side.

19

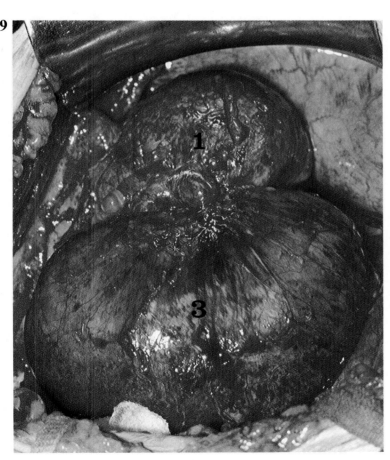

20

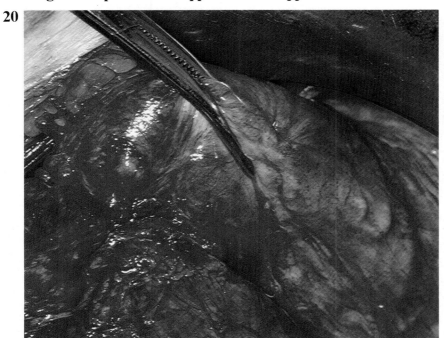

21

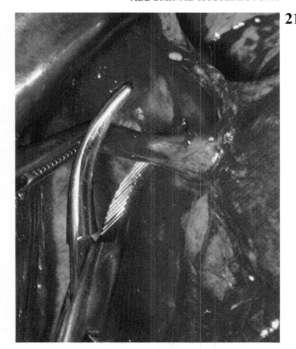

20 to 24 Division of upper uterine attachments

The upper uterine attachments are now clamped and divided. In Figure 20 the broad ligament is clamped and held. In Figure 21 the left round ligament is clamped. In Figure 22 the left infundibulopelvic ligament is clamped and in Figure 23 the right round ligament is secured. In Figure 24 the right infundibulopelvic ligament is ligated.

22

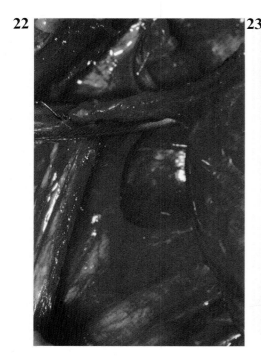

23

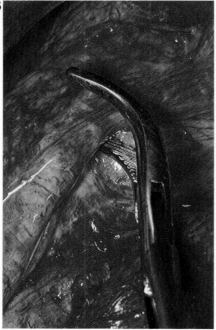

24

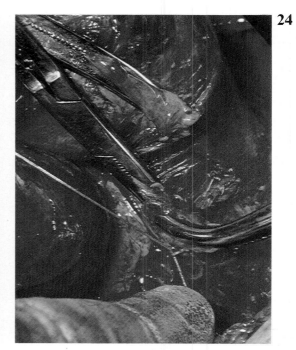

Stage 5: Further definition of ureter

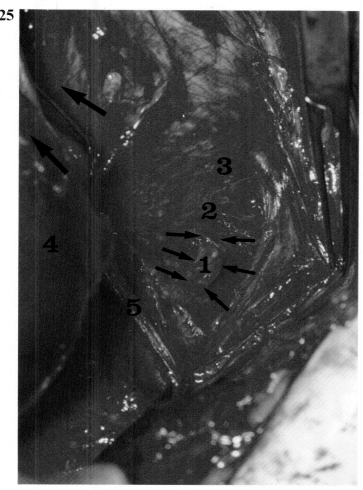

25 Definition and exposure of right ureter

The uterus and appendages are drawn medially (arrowed) and the peritoneal edge held laterally with Allis' forceps to expose the right ureter (1) (outlined) as it approaches the ureteric tunnel (2). The uterine vessels can be seen on the parametrium (3). The relevant structures are: (1) ureter (outlined), (2) ureteric tunnel, (3) uterine vessels, (4) uterus and cystic appendage, (5) peritoneal edge.

26
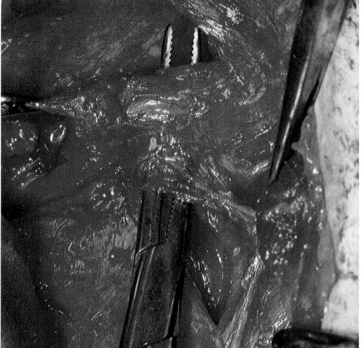

27
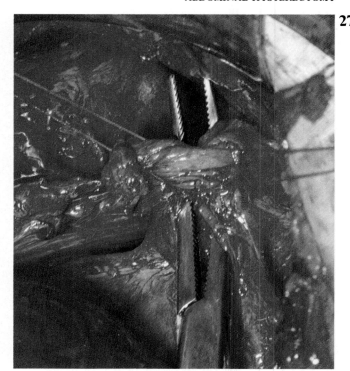

26 to 29 Dividing right uterine vessels to expose ureter

In Figure 26 the forceps have followed the line of the ureter and are opened to display the roof of the tunnel. In Figure 27 the vessels are being tied and in Figure 28 are divided. Figure 29 shows the ureter exposed and being pushed laterally away from the vaginal vault and out of danger; it is outlined.

28
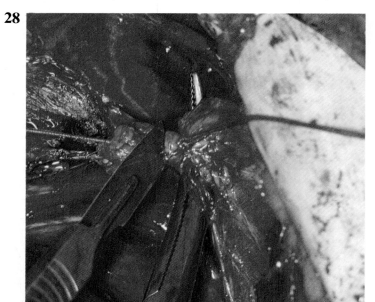

29
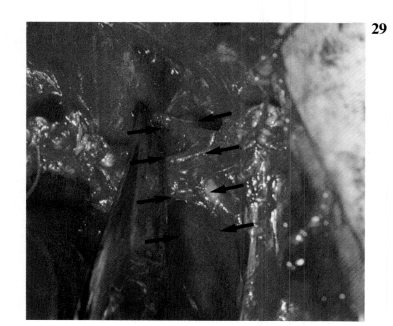

30

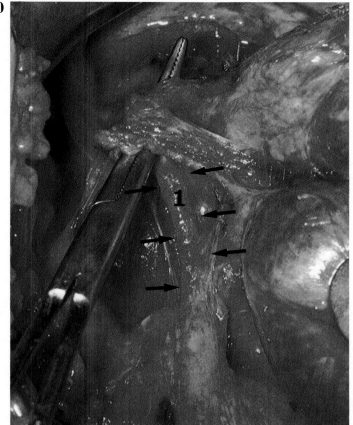

31

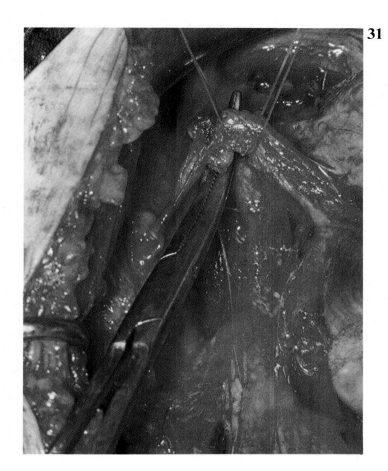

30 to 32 Dividing left uterine vessels to expose ureter

The same procedure is carried out on the left side and the ureter is subsequently displaced laterally out of danger. The ureter (1) is outlined in Figure 30.

32

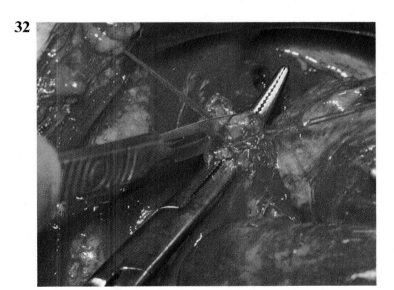

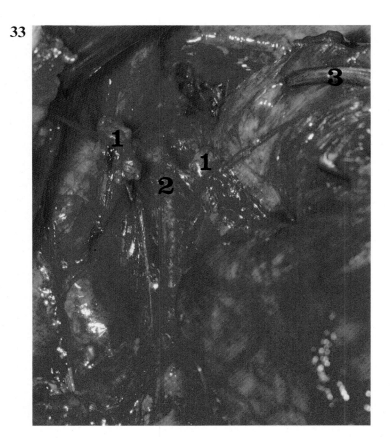

33 and 34 Exposure of left ureter

With the uterine vessels divided at (1) in Figure 33 the ureter (2) is seen running forwards towards the bladder well clear of the uterus which is pulled medially with tissue forceps at (3). In Figure 34 a closer view shows the ureter outlined and expanding as it joins the bladder (4).

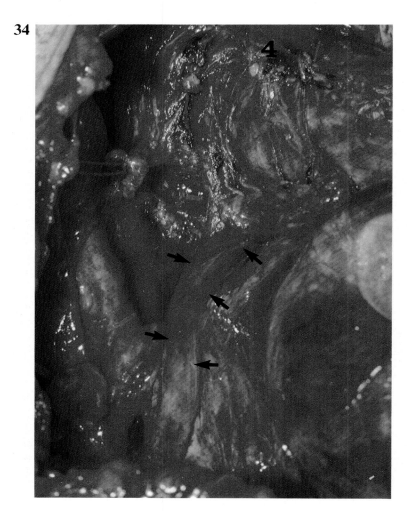

Stage 6: Further mobilisation of deep pelvic appendages

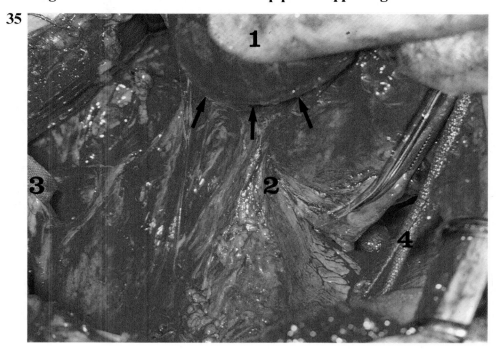

35

35 and 36 Freeing cystic appendages from rectum and pelvic floor

Two stages in the release of the chronically infected appendages are shown. In Figure 35 the cyst is retracted by the surgeon's hand (1) while the rectum (2) will be separated off by blunt dissection and a good plane of separation is

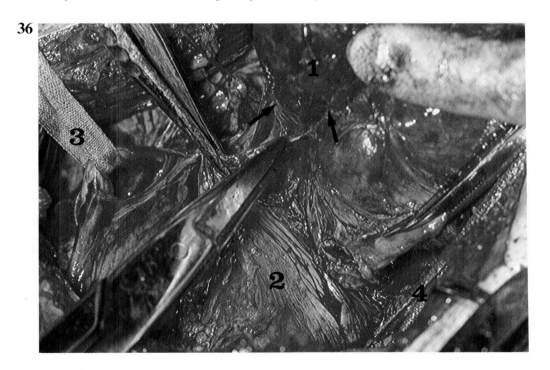

36

developing (arrowed). The possibility of injury to the ureters must be remembered and they have been raised on tapes (3) and (4) so that their exact position is known. In Figure 36 the procedure continues with separation from the pelvic floor centrally. The rectum is now seen to be free. The ureters are still kept in view and the same numerals on the structures apply.

37

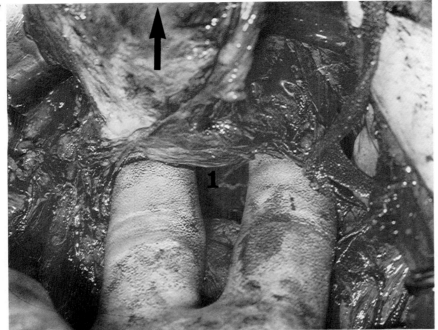

37 Separation of cystic appendages from posterior wall of uterus

With finger dissection the cystic mass is rolled upwards towards the fundus of the uterus as arrowed to expose the posterior wall (1) as far down as the pouch of Douglas. This allows hysterectomy to be completed.

Stage 7: Separation of lower uterine supports

38

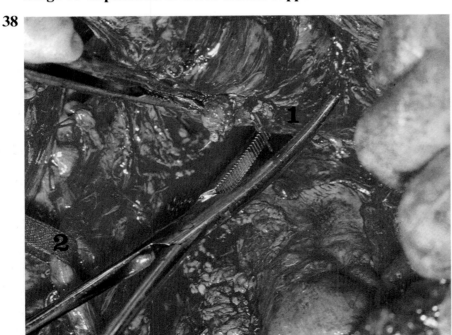

38 Securing right uterosacral ligament

The uterus is still tethered by the uterosacral ligaments (1) in this case and the right ligament is being clamped in the illustration. The left ureter (2) is clearly visible and the position of the other is known to the surgeon and barely seen in the photograph, so that there is no danger to either of the ureters in this situation. It would be perfectly acceptable to divide the ligaments without clamping and use diathermy to seal off any bleeding vessels, but the opportunity is taken here to pinpoint the structures as accurately as possible for demonstration purposes.

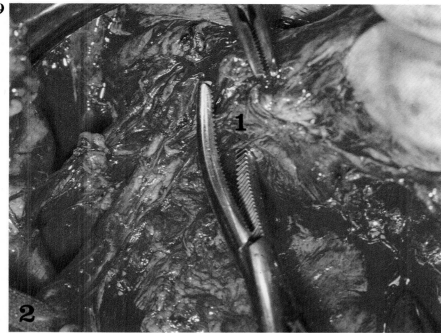

39 Securing left uterosacral ligament

The same procedure as in Figure 38 is carried out on the left side and the left ureter is again visible in the illustration.

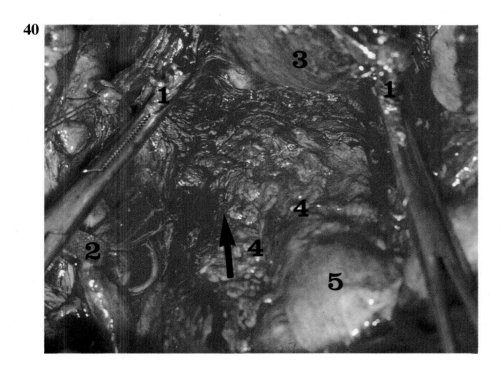

40 Uterus free posteriorly

Forceps (1) and (1) hold the detached uterosacral ligaments and the posterior aspect of the cervix (3) is shown to be quite clear and the pelvic peritoneum (4) separated off and lax over the pouch of Douglas (arrowed). The rectum is more posteriorly at (5). The left ureter is still seen (2).

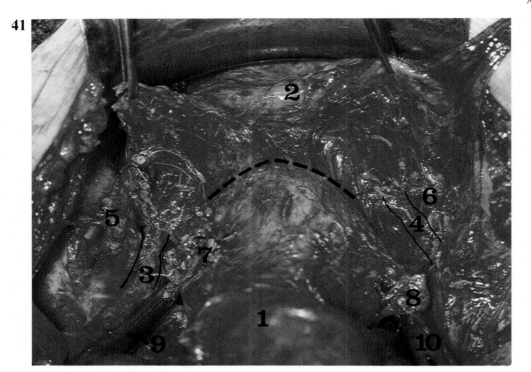

41 Separation of bladder from cervix

The uterus (1) is now drawn back in retroposition to show the bladder (2) anteriorly and the line of separation between them (broken line). Both ureters are outlined (3) and (4) with the ligated uterine pedicles lateral to them (5) and (6). The distal ends of the uterine vessels are seen (7) and (8) and the forceps (9) and (10) hold the cut uterosacral ligaments.

Stage 8: Removal of uterus

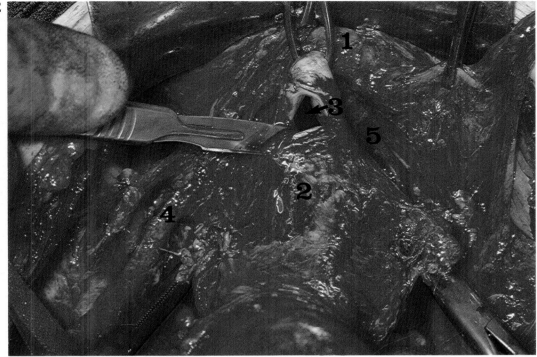

42 Removal of uterus (1)

Having separated the bladder (1) well down off the cervix (2) and having defined the lower limit of the cervix with finger and thumb an incision is made through the anterior vaginal wall with the scalpel as shown at (3). The ureters are still visible (4) and (5).

43

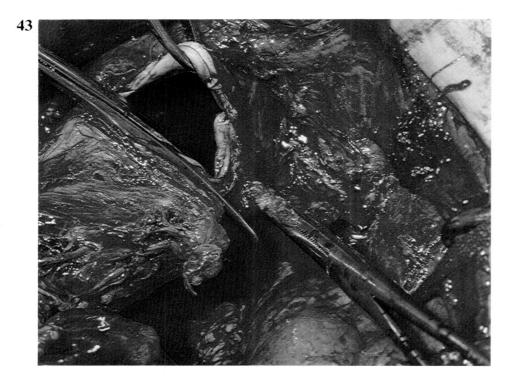

43 and 44 Removal of uterus (2)

First on the right side in Figure 43 and then on the left side in
Figure 44 the scissors open up the vaginal vault anteriorly in
removing the uterus with a generous cuff of vagina. The
forceps are still seen on the uterosacral ligaments.

44

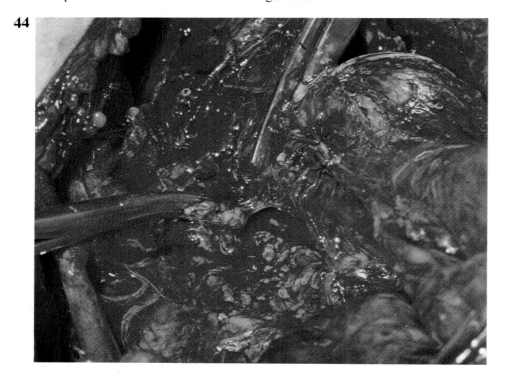

45

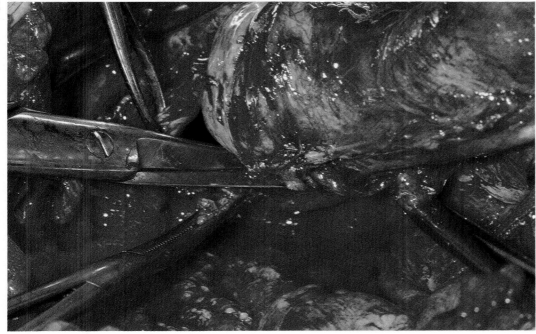

45 and 46 Removal of uterus (3)

The process of removal continues posteriorly on the left in Figure 45 and on the right in Figure 46. The uterosacral forceps are still in position and the ureters are still visible on their tapes.

46

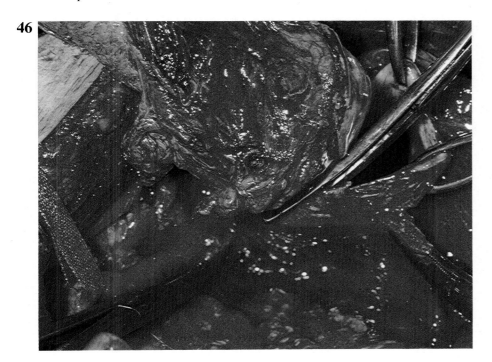

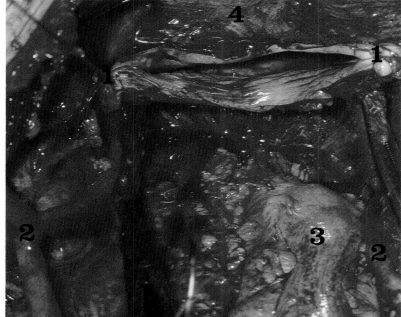

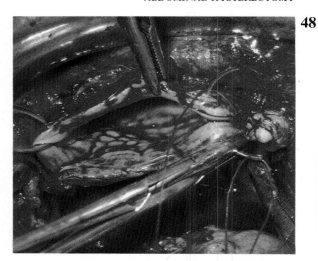

47 and 48 Closure of vaginal vault

The very wide vaginal vault is seen in Figure 47 with lateral sutures inserted (1). Closure of the vault with a series of mattress sutures is about to begin. Both ureters (2), rectum (3) and bladder (4) are seen and the forceps are still on the uterosacral ligaments. The ends of the uterosacral ligaments will be incorporated into the vaginal vault during closure by the mattress sutures to give additional support. The mattress suture on the right side of the vault is on its outward journey in Figure 48 and will pick up the uterosacral ligament on its return.

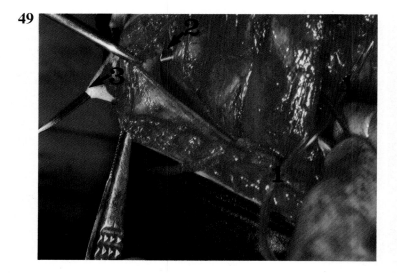

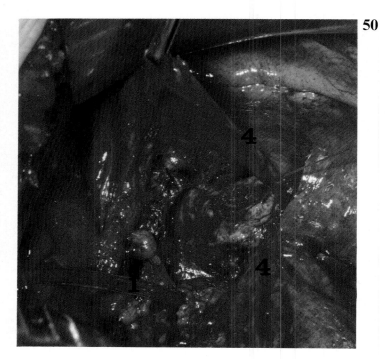

49 and 50 Drainage of pelvis

In Figure 49 a Redivac drain (1) is being placed on the patient's left side with the pilot trochar needle coming through the peritoneum lateral to the rectus muscle (2) and emerging through the skin lateral to the wound (3). Figure 50 shows the intrapelvic view of the same drain (1) emerging from under the peritoneum (4) which is being sutured. The drain extends across the pelvic floor and vaginal vault under the peritoneum and is placed carefully in position before the peritoneum is closed. One such drain is usually sufficient but some surgeons prefer to have a drain crossing the pelvis from each side.

51

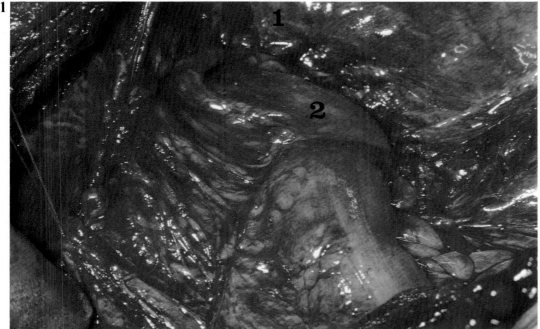

51 Closure of peritoneum complete

The pelvic floor has been completely covered with peritoneum along the line between bladder (1) and rectum (2). The tissues are under no tension, the wound is obviously dry and the Redivac drains are *in situ*. Care was taken to keep the ureters in view while approximating the peritoneal edges.

52

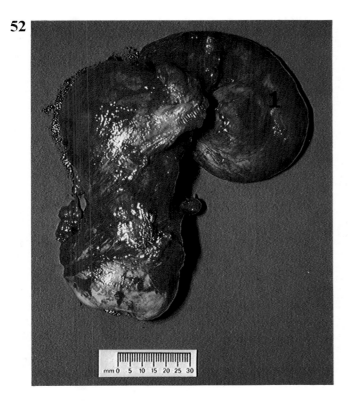

52 Operation specimen

The large cystic mass (1) is seen adherant to the posterior-superior aspect of the uterine body. Note the lack of induration around the cervix and vaginal vault attachment.

Conditions demanding modification of basic hysterectomy technique: accompanying vaginal vault prolapse

Those who consider vaginal rather than abdominal hysterectomy the normal procedure will see little need for this operation. However, unless the surgeon is skilled in vaginal hysterectomy there are several situations where it is required. In the case used for illustration there was a huge mass of fibroids that could only have been removed vaginally by morcellement; this was accompanied by a lax vaginal vault above a narrow and previously repaired prolapse of the vaginal walls. Less rarely the uterus is merely very large, is adherent in the pelvis or there is accompanying ovarian pathology. Occasionally a patient having hysterectomy has vault laxity but well supported vaginal walls. There is no doubt that many able surgeons are not prepared to risk the known morbidity of vaginal hysterectomy when the main object of removing the uterus can be done more safely via the abdomen.

The procedure described is straightforward and in essence involves the removal of a V-shaped wedge from the upper end of the anterior and posterior vaginal walls. The narrowed vault is closed in the sagittal rather than the coronal plane and is supported not only by the uterosacral but also by the round ligaments as will be shown in the illustrations.

If the surgeon proceeds to repair the lower vagina after this procedure, he will be surprised not only at the excellence of the vault repair but also at its extent when seen from below. Only the lower part of the vagina still requires operation.

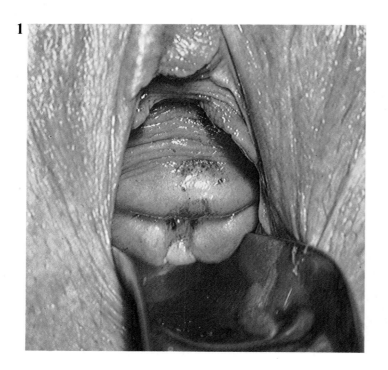

1 Vaginal view of vault prolapse
The cervix descends to the introitus although the lower vaginal walls are well supported and the perineum is intact.

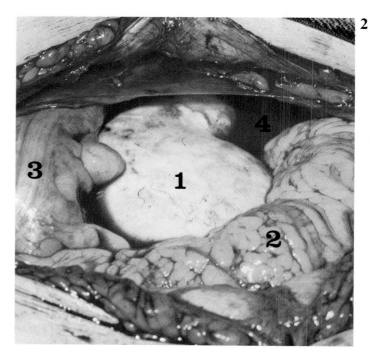

2 General view on opening abdomen
A large pedunculated fibroid is seen in the centre of the wound (1) with the omentum (2) in the upper part of the wound and the descending colon (3) on the left. There were multiple intramural and pedunculated fibroids. There is free fluid (4) in the peritoneum also.

Stage 1: Separation of lower uterine supports

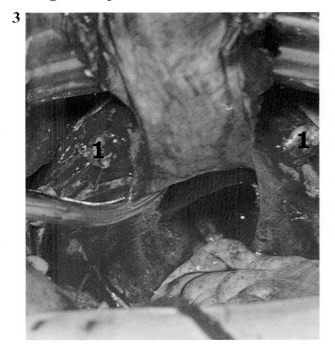

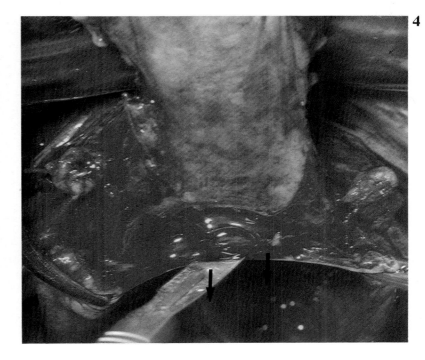

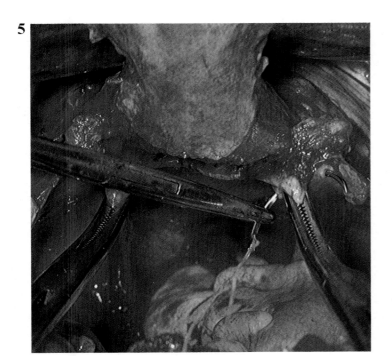

3 to 5 Securing uterosacral ligaments

The hysterectomy has proceeded as far as ligation of the uterine vessels (1). The uterosacral ligaments are on the stretch in Figure 3 with the left being clamped. In Figure 4 both uterosacral ligaments have been detached and the peritoneum between is being incised and pushed down in the direction of the arrows. In Figure 5 the right ligament is being transfixed before ligation which is then completed on both sides.

6

7

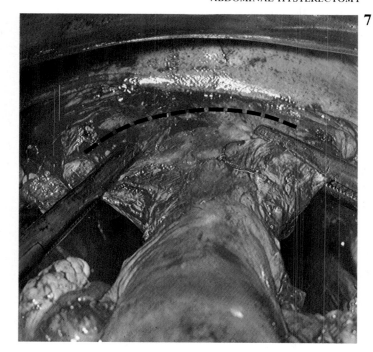

6 and 7 Securing vaginal angles

The level of the external os in the vagina is marked by the stitch on the anterior aspect of the vault in the illustrations and shows that the vault is both wide and lax. In Figure 6 the left vaginal angle is clamped well down on the vagina and in Figure 7 this is repeated on the other side. The outline of the bladder attachments is seen as a broken line.

8

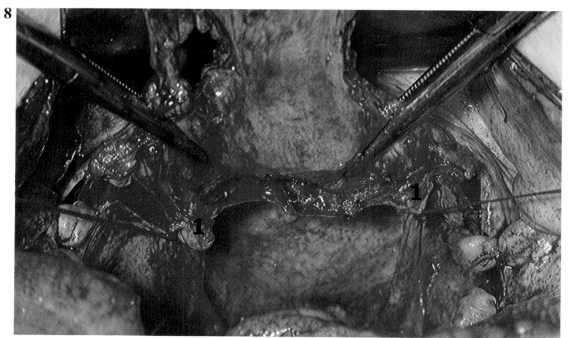

8 Posterior view of wide vaginal vault

It will be seen that there is a fairly wide area of redundant vault tissue. The two clamps are attached to the vaginal angles; the cut and ligated uterosacral ligaments are seen (1).

Stage 2: Opening and refashioning of vaginal vault

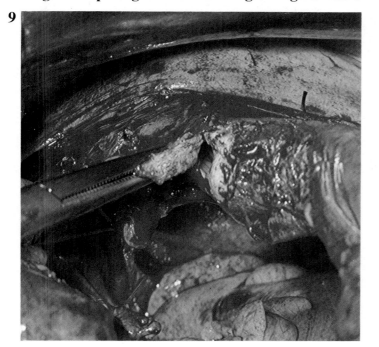

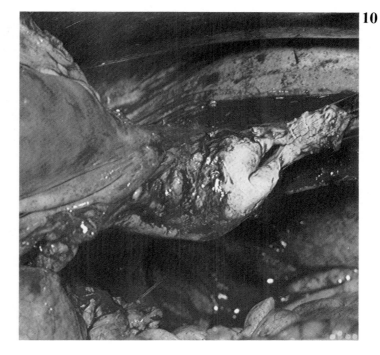

9 Opening vaginal vault (left)

The angle of the vagina has been opened medial to the forceps which also hold the cardinal ligament; the level is seen to be below the stitch which indicates the level of the external cervical os. The vagina is not opened wide on purpose, so that the excess tissue to be removed remains attached to the uterus and is easily defined as it is held on the stretch.

10 Opening vaginal vault (right)

The same procedure as in Figure 9 is carried out on the right side. The aim in these steps of the operation is to allow entry of the scissors on each side, so that the correct amount of excess tissue can be excised.

11

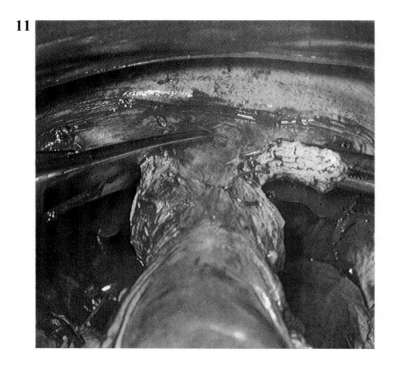

12

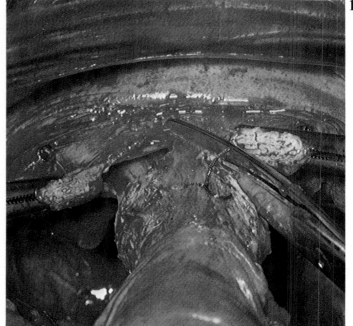

11 to 14 V-excision of anterior vaginal wall at vault

In Figure 11 the scissors cut down and medially towards the midline to make the left limb of a V-shaped incision. In Figure 12 the same is done on the opposite side removing the central excess tissue. In Figure 13 the anterior vaginal wall is transfixed at the apex of the V with a PGA No. 1 suture. In Figure 14 the suture has been tied.

13

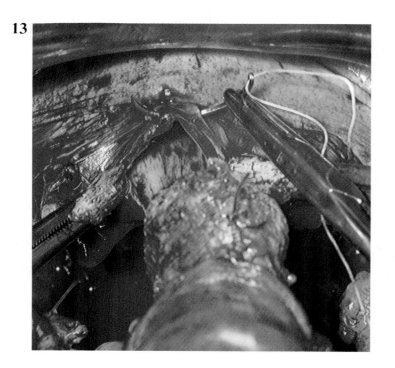

14

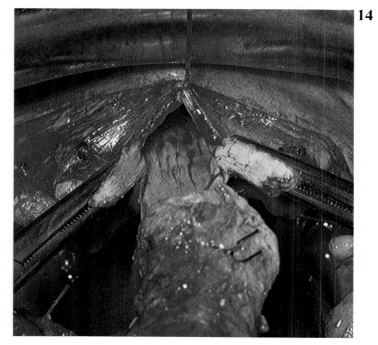

15

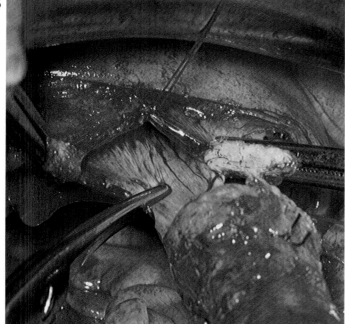

16

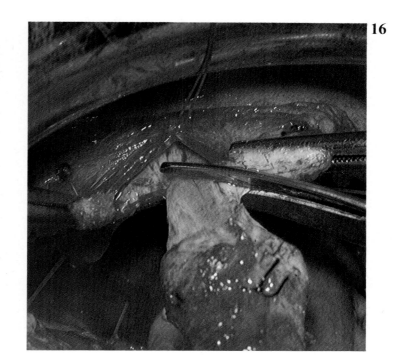

15 to 17 V-excision of posterior vaginal wall at vault

A similar procedure is followed on the posterior aspect. In Figure 15 the left limb of the V is cut and in Figure 16 the right limb of the V is cut. Figure 17 shows the uterus removed and a posterior stitch being placed at the apex of the V.

17

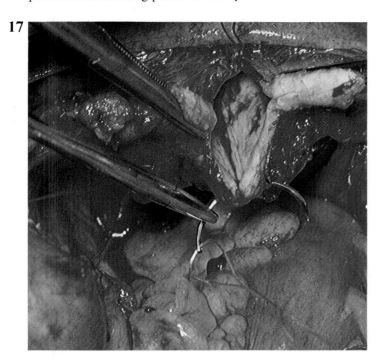

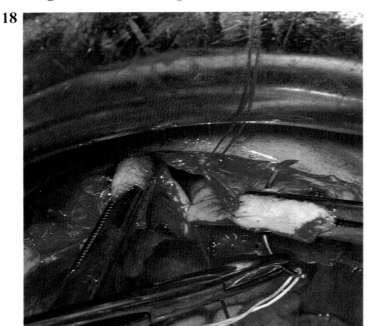

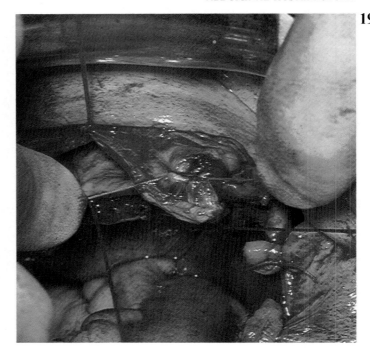

18 and 19 Closure of right lateral angle of the vaginal vault
The vaginal angle where the forceps also include in their grasp the inner end of the cardinal ligament is transfixed in Figure 18 and then tied in the usual way in Figure 19.

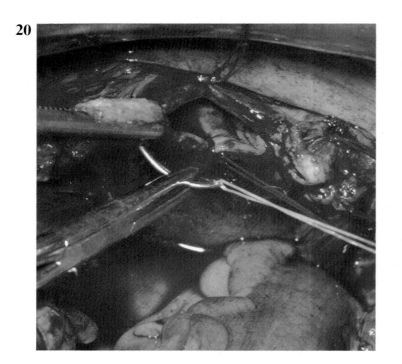

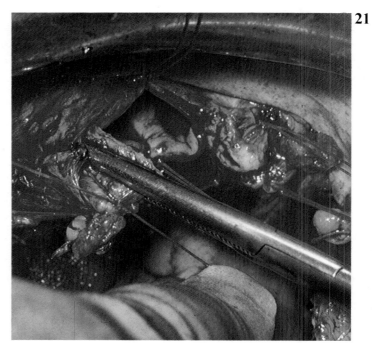

20 and 21 Closure of left lateral angle of the vaginal vault
The same procedure is carried out on the left side.

Stage 4: Approximation of uterosacral ligaments

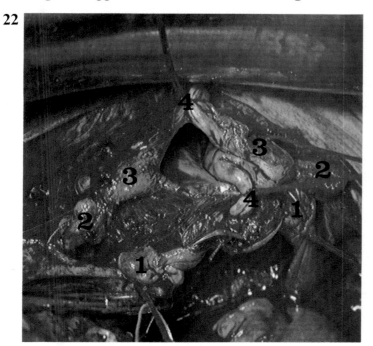

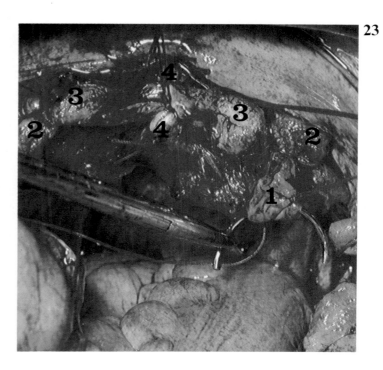

23

22 and 23 Approximation of uterosacral ligaments (1)

It is important that the uterosacral ligaments be brought together closely to support the vault; the illustrations show the first step or outward journey of the needle carrying the suture. In Figure 22 the left uterosacral ligament is transfixed and in Figure 23 the right also. A good bite of tissue is taken. Numbers indicate the structures thus: uterosacral ligaments (1), uterine pedicles (2), vaginal angles (3), anterior and posterior V closure of vault (4).

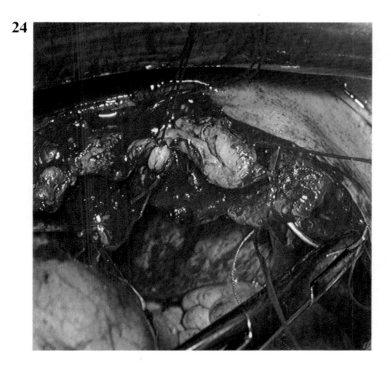

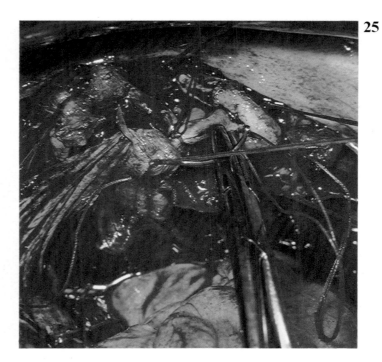

24 and 25 Approximation of uterosacral ligaments (2)

The return journey of the suture carrying needle is shown. In Figure 24 a second bite is taken to encircle the right ligament and in Figure 25 the same method is used to encircle the left ligament, so that when the ends of the stitch are tied the pedicles will be fixed together firmly. A transverse mattress suture is in fact being used to fix the uterosacral ligaments together.

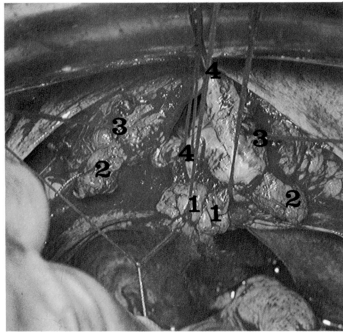

26 Approximation of uterosacral ligaments (3)
The suture is seen being tied firmly to approximate the uterosacral ligaments and form a firm posterior border to the vaginal vault. This is a very important stitch and should be placed accurately. The structures are numbered as in Figures 22 and 23.

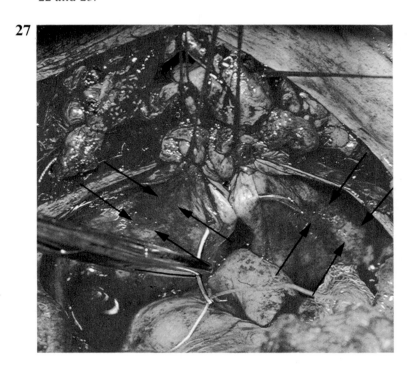

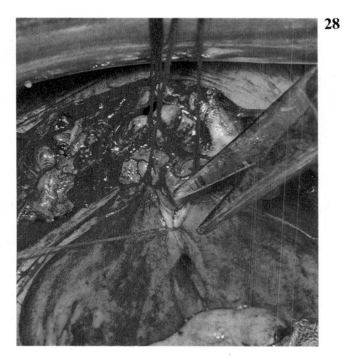

27 and 28 Further approximation of uterosacral ligaments
It is desirable to close the pouch of Douglas further back and prevent subsequent enterocoele. In Figure 27 the needle pierces both ligaments in turn; in Figure 28 these are drawn together closely and a stitch is being cut. The pouch of Douglas is now almost non-existent. It might be asked if there is any danger of damage to the ureters by such a vault closure. The ureters are well lateral to the uterosacral ligaments and are quite safe as long as the ligaments are transfixed with the stitch and not encircled widely. The position of the ureters is outlined by arrows.

Stage 5: Completion of vaginal vault closure

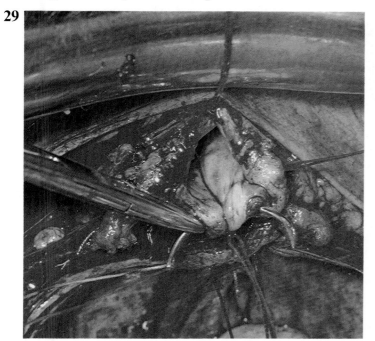

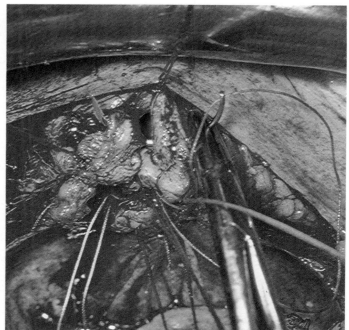

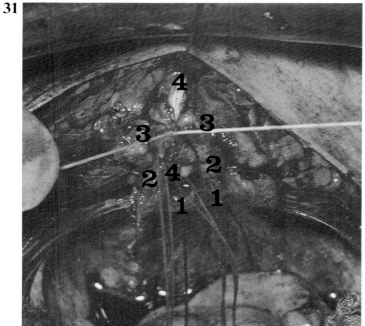

29 to 31 Closure of centre of vaginal vault

The vaginal vault is in fact closed anteroposteriorly instead of transversely as is usual; it is this fact which accounts for its subsequent strength and support. A strong transverse mattress suture which encircles the cardinal ligaments at the vaginal angles is used to effect this and the steps in placing it are shown in the illustrations. In Figure 29 the two limbs of the posterior V have been transfixed from left to right. In Figure 30 the suture has gone round the right ligated angle with its included cardinal ligament and is traversing the limbs of the anterior V. In Figure 31 the suture has encircled the left angle and cardinal ligament pedicle and is being tied to close the whole vault in an anteroposterior plane. Numbers indicate the structures: uterosacral ligaments (1), uterine pedicles (2), vaginal angles (3), anterior and posterior V closure of vault (4).

32

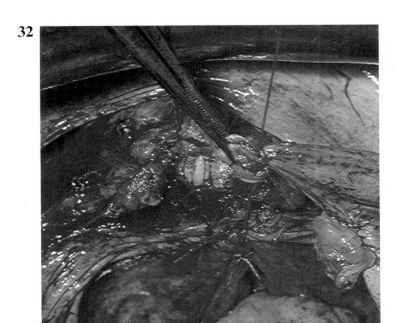

33

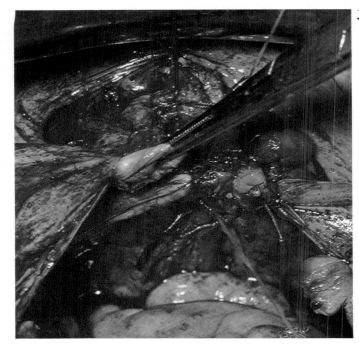

32 to 34 Incorporation of round ligaments in the vault

It is usual to stitch the ends of the round ligaments to the vaginal vault to give maximum support in such cases and that is shown here. In Figure 32 the right round ligament has been drawn medially and is being tied in place by a suture which transfixes the vault on that side. In Figure 33 the left ligament is being drawn in to be tied to the vault in the same way; in Figure 34 both ligaments are shown in their new position.

34

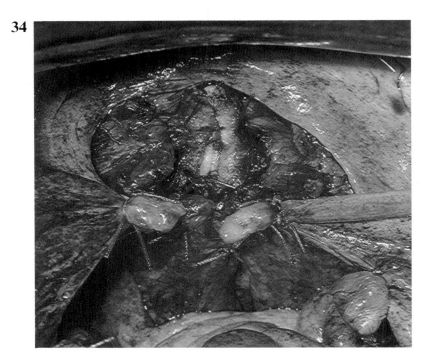

35

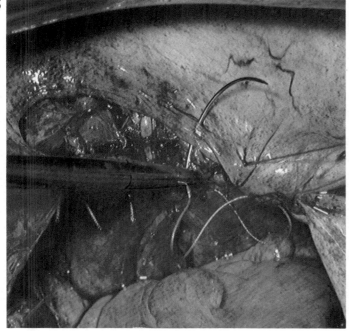

36

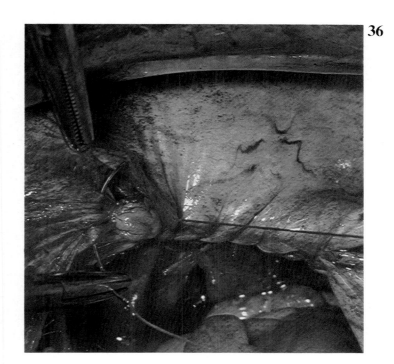

35 to 37 Closure of pelvic peritoneum

In Figure 35 the pedicles in the right angle of the pelvic wound have been buried and the stitch is proceeding across the pelvis. In Figure 36 the left-sided pedicles are being covered and in Figure 37 the pelvic floor is completely invested with peritoneum.

37

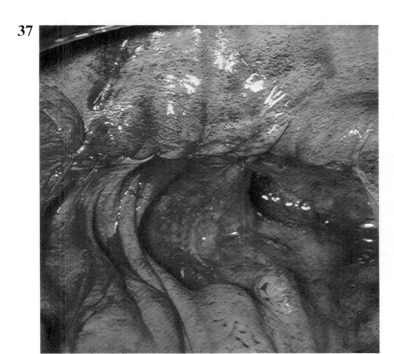

38

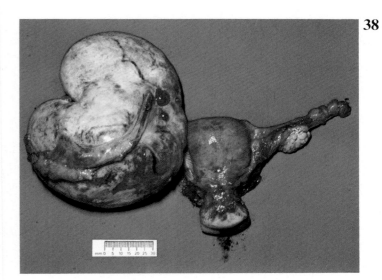

38 Specimen

The uterus with its large pedunculated fibroid is shown. The V-shaped excised portions of the vaginal wall are still attached to the uterus.

Conditions demanding modification of basic hysterectomy technique: supravaginal (subtotal) hysterectomy

This operation is not recommended nor is it a procedure which a trained gynaecologist would normally use. It is included in the Atlas because in certain unusual circumstances it may be the safest thing to do and that is discussed below.

No attempt is made to catalogue the disadvantages of the operation; suffice to say that the cervix has no supportive function at the vault of the vagina and no lubricant action in coitus as was at one time thought. Thus there is no reason for its retention. The case for its removal is even stronger and is based on statistics which show that the incidence of cancer of the cervical stump is unacceptably high.

The authors expect that among their readers will be some who are relatively inexperienced in surgery and some who are experienced in general surgery but not in gynaecological techniques. There are circumstances where it might be life-saving for such doctors to remove the uterus, provided time and blood were not lost in an inexperienced attempt to remove the cervix also. It needs little imagination to conjure up various combinations of circumstance which might arise from the factors of anaemia and poor general condition, lack

of blood for transfusion, poor anaesthesia, inadequate assistance and no immediate recourse to the facilities we accept daily as normal.

The practice of gynaecological surgery is not so sophisticated and excellent that experienced surgeons do not sometimes elect to do a sub-total hysterectomy for very sound reasons. In most such instances they would subsequently remove the cervical stump; such a procedure is included in the Atlas. The special circumstances might include a very large mass of fibroids associated with an elongated cervix where access to the region of the vault is very difficult. Supravaginal hysterectomy followed by removal of the cervical stump is probably the safest procedure in these circumstances. In cases of chronic endometriosis with multiple firm pelvic adhesions, we have seen the most experienced pelvic surgeons accept a sub-total hysterectomy as the safest if not the best they can achieve in adverse circumstances. In obstetrics, and unless the surgeon is experienced, caesarean hysterectomy is more likely and probably more safely done as a sub-total procedure.

Stage 1: Separation of bladder from cervix

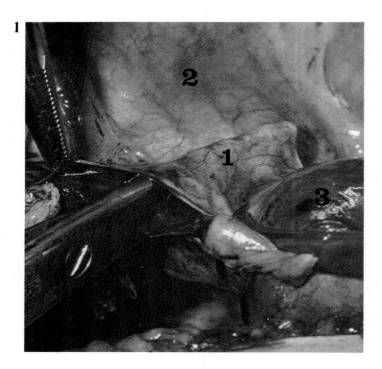

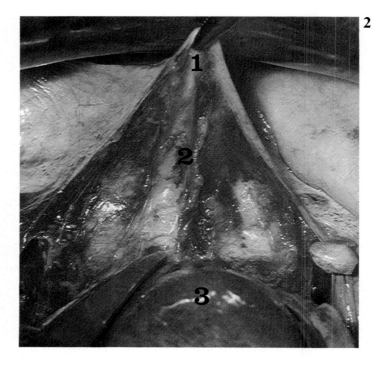

1 Definition of uterovesical pouch
The peritoneum (1) between the bladder (2) and the uterus (3) is raised before its division.

2 Separation of bladder from cervix
With the centre of the peritoneal fold held in dissecting forceps (1) the scissors separate the bladder (2) from the uterus (3) working close to the latter until a plane of separation is found.

Stage 2: Defining and securing uterine vessels

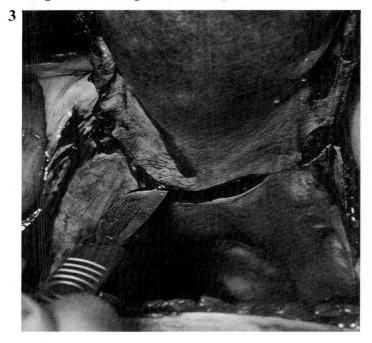

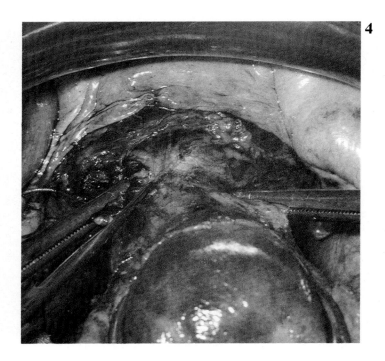

3 Opening posterior layer of broad ligament
The posterior layer of the broad ligament has been opened on each side; the peritoneum between the uterosacral ligaments is being divided with the scalpel to allow access to the region of the isthmus of the uterus.

4 Securing and detaching uterine pedicles
Both uterine pedicles have been clamped and the left is being detached with scissors.

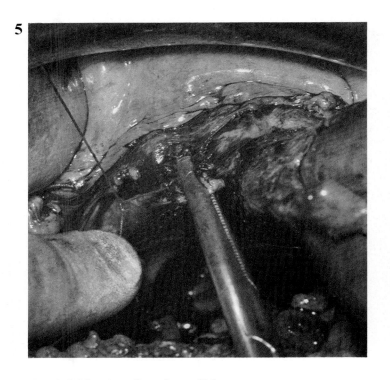

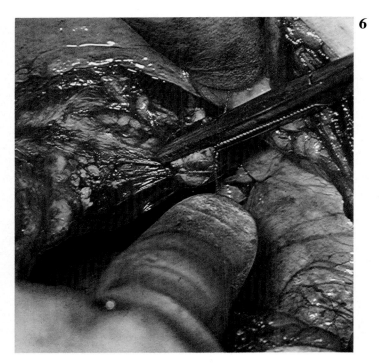

5 and 6 Ligation of uterine pedicles
The left pedicle is being ligated in Figure 5; the right pedicle is being ligated in Figure 6.

7

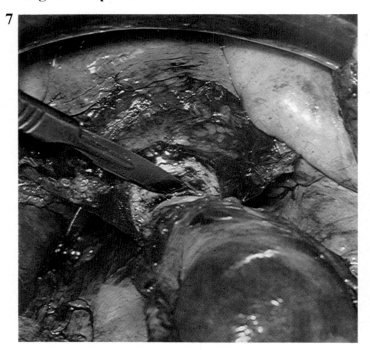

8

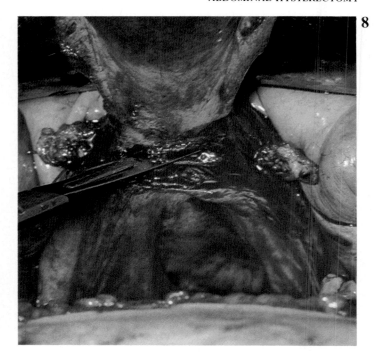

7 to 10 Amputation of uterus from the cervix

With the body of the uterus retracted posteriorly the scalpel commences separation anteriorly in Figure 7 and cuts to the depth of the upper cervical canal. In Figure 8 the uterus is lifted forwards and the same procedure is continued posteriorly. This is continued in Figure 9; in Figure 10 the uterus is again retracted to allow complete severance from the cervix. When sub-total hysterectomy was a common operation it was generally advised that one should cut slightly downwards to give the effect of 'coning-out' the uterus, both to excise the maximum amount of cervical epithelium and also to allow neater closure of the cervical stump.

9

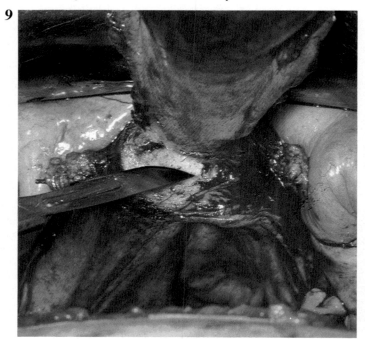

10

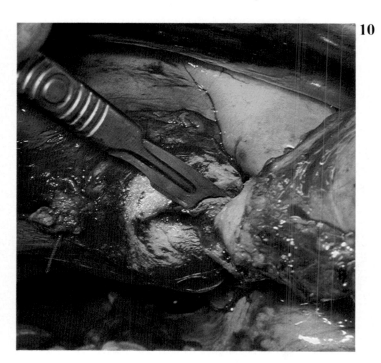

Stage 4: Closure of cervical stump

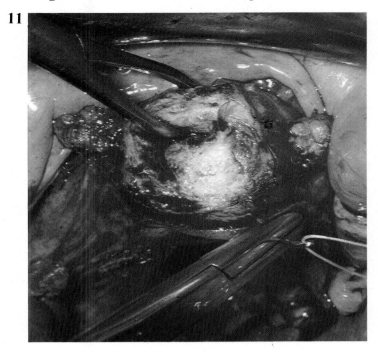

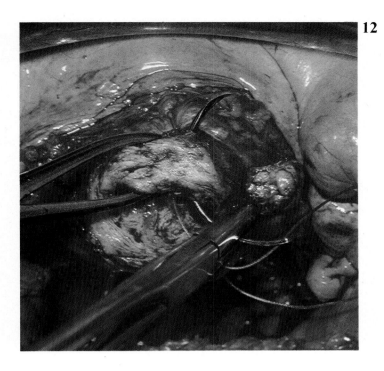

11 to 14 Closure of upper end of cervix (1)

The various steps in closing the upper end of the cervix are illustrated. In Figure 11 the posterior lip is taken up on a cutting needle carrying a PGA No. 1 suture and in Figure 12 the anterior lip is pierced at the corresponding point. Figure 13 shows the stitch tied and the 'coning' effect of the amputation allows neat apposition of the edges. A similar suture has been placed on the left side in Figure 14.

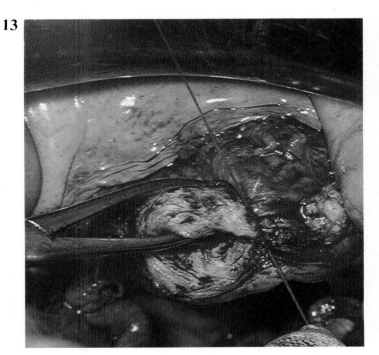

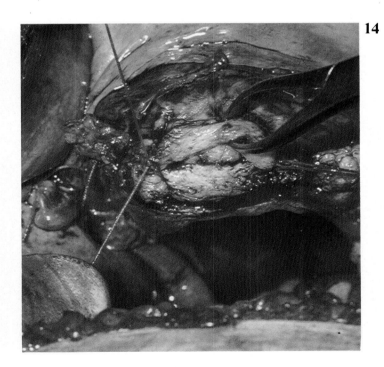

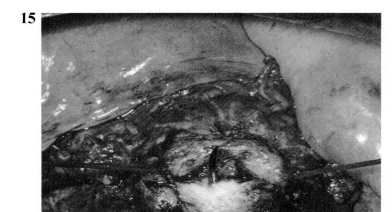

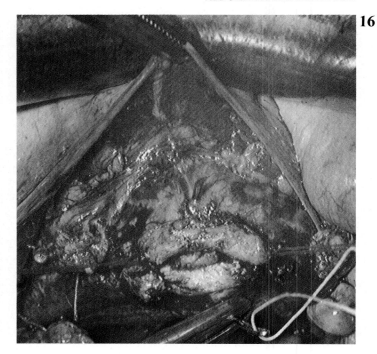

15 and 16 Closure of upper end of cervix (2)

The process of closure continues in the illustrations. In Figure 15 the posterior lip is again taken up centrally; in Figure 16 the needle proceeds to take up the anterior lip at the corresponding point.

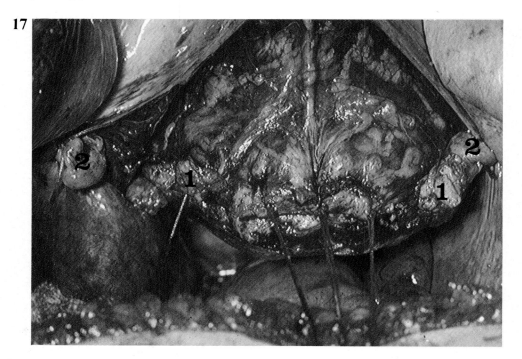

17 Closure of cervix completed

The cervix is shown neatly closed and held up by the uncut sutures. The uterine pedicles (1) and the round ligament pedicles (2) are seen.

Stage 5: Closure of pelvic peritoneum

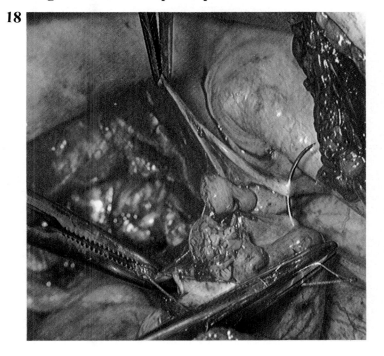

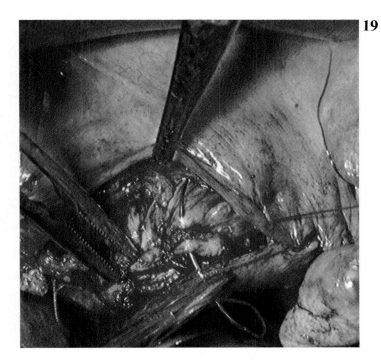

18 to 20 Closure of pelvic peritoneum

Stages in approximation of the pelvic peritoneum are shown. In Figure 18 the right pedicles are about to be covered by the half purse-string suture being placed. In Figure 19 the stitch proceeds across the cervical stump and is attached to it by occasional stitches to eliminate dead space. In Figure 20 the peritoneum is shown completely closed.

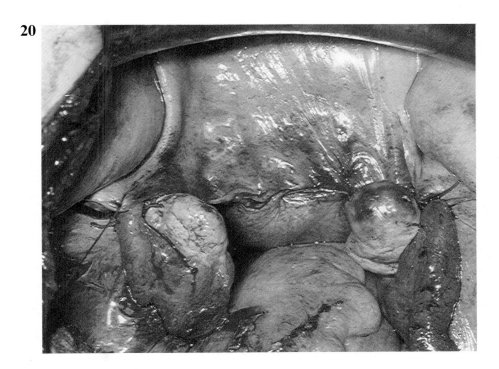

Removal of residual cervix

The operation described below is applicable where the uterus has been removed by cutting across the region of the isthmus and where it is considered essential to remove the remaining cervix. Possible reasons for undertaking such a series of procedures are touched on in the introduction to sub-total hysterectomy (page 154). In essence, a bulky and awkward uterus has been removed supravaginally, subsequently allowing access to the cervix which is excised in the manner now described.

Removal of the cervix at a later date as a prophylactic or curative procedure can also be carried out vaginally; in the latter instance the operation presents no particular difficulties.

Because this operation consists of a number of small individual manoeuvres it has not been divided into definitive stages.

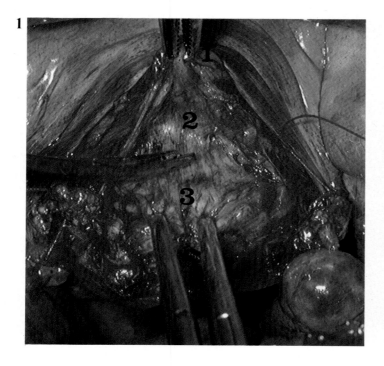

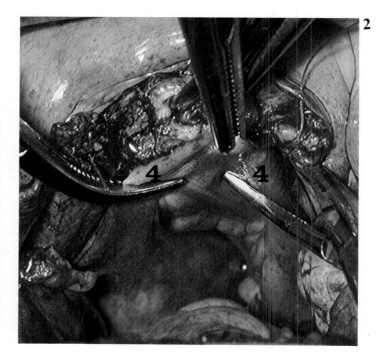

1 Separation of bladder from cervix

The peritoneum (1) is held upwards by the dissecting forceps while the scissors separate the bladder (2) from the anterior aspect of the cervix (3). The latter is held up by the tissue forceps.

2 Securing uterosacral ligaments

The uterosacral ligaments (4) have not been detached in a sub-total hysterectomy and must now be clamped before separation.

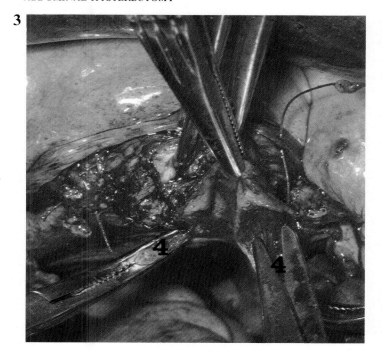

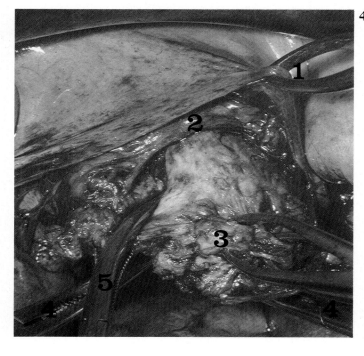

3 Detaching uterosacral ligaments

Detaching the uterosacral ligaments is done with scissors as shown and the pedicles may be tied or the forceps left attached as in this case (4) and (4).

4 and 5 Clamping vaginal angles

The cervix (3) is lifted up by the attached tissue forceps and with the forceps (1) on the peritoneum and holding the bladder (2) well clear, the vaginal angles are clamped on the left in Figure 4 and on the right in Figure 5 by forceps (5).

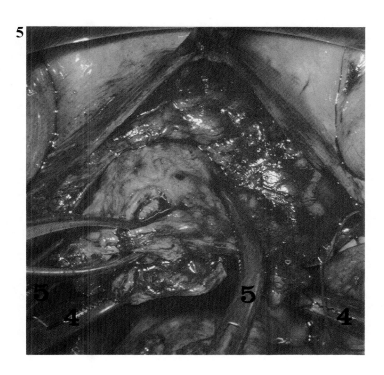

6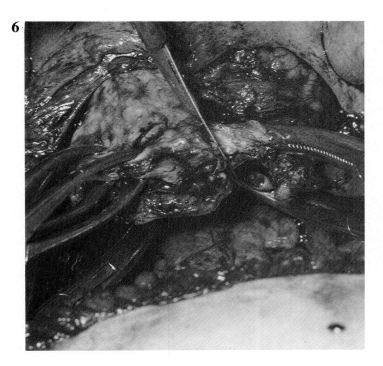

7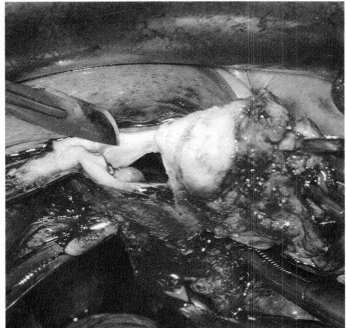

6 to 8 Removal of cervical stump

The vaginal vault is opened on the right side in Figure 6, on the left in Figure 7, and the scissors cut the anterior vaginal wall in Figure 8. It only remains to divide the posterior wall attachment and the cervix is free.

8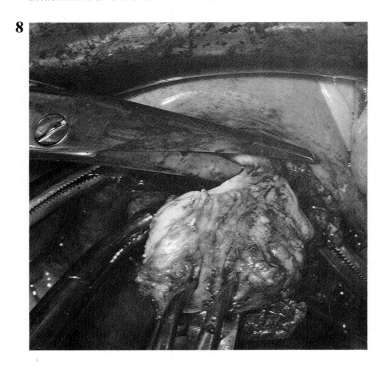

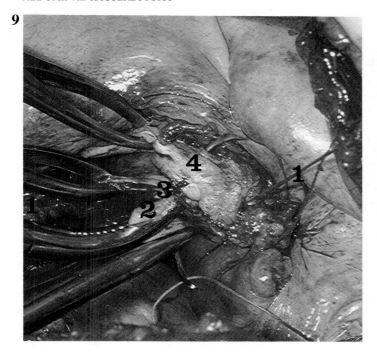

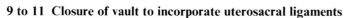

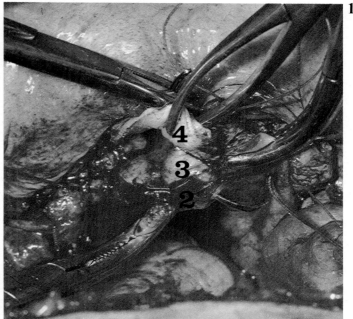

9 to 11 Closure of vault to incorporate uterosacral ligaments

The vaginal angles have been ligated and in Figure 9 the uncut suture on the right side is numbered (1). That on the left can just be seen (1). The needle carrying the suture which is being inserted has transfixed the right uterosacral ligament (2) and has completed its outward journey through both posterior and anterior vaginal walls (3) and (4). In Figure 10 the suture makes the return journey through the anterior and posterior vaginal walls in turn (4) and (3) and again picks up the uterosacral ligament (2) to enclose it in the ligature. In Figure 11 the ligature is being run up tight to close the right side of the vaginal vault. The same procedure is then followed on the left side.

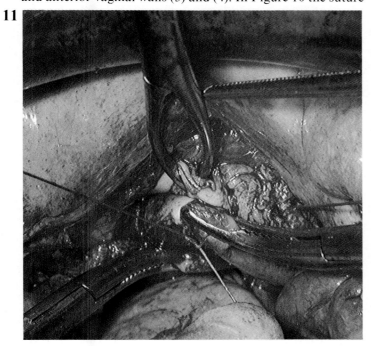

12

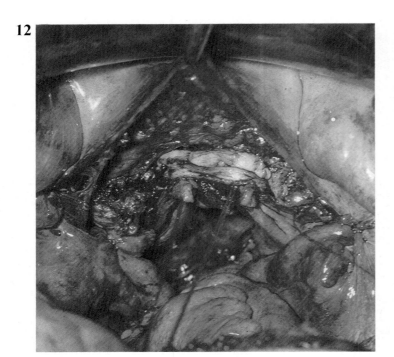

13

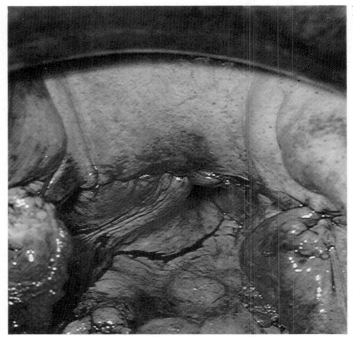

12 Vault of vagina closed

The photograph shows the vaginal vault closed. The two long sutures are those described in Figures 9, 10 and 11 and it will be seen that they have attached the uterosacral ligament firmly to the vaginal vault.

13 Closure of pelvic peritoneum completed

The appearance after removal of the cervical stump is shown with a neat and dry closure of the pelvic peritoneum.

4: Myomectomy

Myomectomy may be the treatment of choice for women of childbearing age with symptoms related to uterine myomota (fibroids). The usual reason for doing this operation is to preserve the uterus and safeguard future fertility, although social and religious prejudices may also be major influences. Where subsequent fertility need not be considered hysterectomy is, in many ways, a more satisfactory alternative and is attended by fewer complications.

If there are clear indications for myomectomy and the operation goes according to plan, it can be a very satisfying procedure for patient and doctor in that it relieves symptoms without prejudice to fertility. It may even inadvertently or by expectation actually increase fertility. However, more often than not the prospects of operative success are less predictable with doubts about what the surgeon may find when he opens the abdomen and what he may be able to achieve. Ordinary prudence demands a very cautious approach to all such cases.

Patients have to be advised that myomectomy in any individual case may prove to be technically impossible or if persevered with may be dangerous and leave a much weakened uterus which could give rise to complications in a future pregnancy and labour. In such circumstances the surgeon must have permission to proceed to hysterectomy if he feels that safety demands such a course. Patients will sometimes evince shocked surprise that such unwelcome possibilities have to be raised and subsequent discussion can be uncomfortable. However, these matters cannot be glossed over. The authors consider it very important that the doctor and patient fully understand each other.

When women married later than at present, they frequently presented in their mid-thirties suffering from fibroids and at the same time were desperately keen to have a child. Myomectomy was indicated and was a popular operation but often practised to ingenuous extremes in an attempt to remove even the tiniest fibroid. Shelling out numerous fibroids requires no great degree of surgical skill but it greatly weakens the uterus and inevitably leads to haematomata. The concept is mistaken because no matter how thorough the surgery, some seedling fibroids will be missed and will grow. Meanwhile they will not prejudice fertility and can be ignored. The aim should be to remove those fibroids which are believed to be causing menorrhagia, infertility or risks in pregnancy and to do so with minimal trauma and morbidity. We believe that this point of view is now generally accepted.

At operation the thoughtful surgeon examines the uterus carefully after opening the abdomen but before embarking on myomectomy. It is preferable to incise the wall of the uterus at points adjacent to or underlying loose peritoneum, so that the muscle incision can be covered with peritoneum; this can often be planned once it has been established where the larger fibroids lie. It is of considerable benefit to the patient if two or more fibroids can be removed through the same muscle incision by tunnelling laterally from the cavity of the first fibroid removed; such a procedure may also be planned in advance after a careful examination.

Surgical technique is obviously very important. A primary principle is gentle enucleation of the fibroids from their capsules through incisions of minimal length. When removing an intramural fibroid it is essential to see that the cavity of the uterus is opened, both to allow exploration for fibroids presenting into the cavity and to establish a safe drainage exit for blood oozing from the site of the fibroid. The fibroid cavities themselves are always carefully closed by building up the requisite number of muscle layers, so that there is no dead space. PGA No. 0 suture is strong enough and should also be used as sparingly as possible, because the addition of any excess foreign body suture material added to the inevitable haematomata make up a likely recipe for serous and possible infected collections. The surface peritoneum should be approximated neatly to avoid adhesion to omentum or bowel.

Despite the undoubted short-term advantages of a judicious myomectomy operation, follow-up of these patients over a number of years shows that even if a pregnancy or pregnancies supervene, further fibroids nearly always develop. The surgeon finds himself eventually removing an irregularly enlarged uterus to relieve menorrhagia.

Removal of a single posterior fibroid

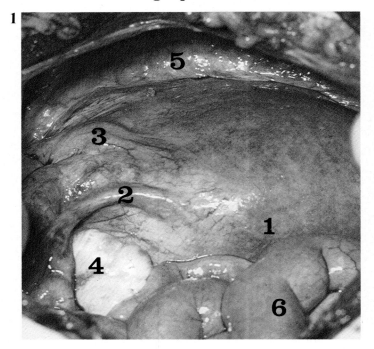

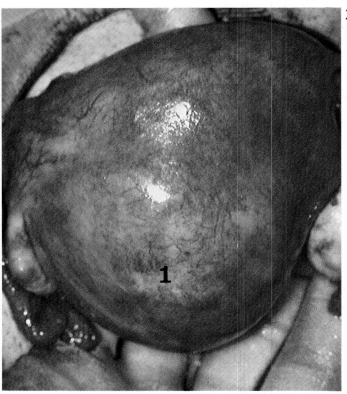

There is only one fibroid of any size in this case and that is on the posterolateral wall. Its removal allows demonstration of the essential steps in myomectomy where adjacent loose peritoneum is not available.

1 General view on opening abdomen

In this case the uterus is seen to be generally enlarged with a fibroid on the left side posteriorly (1). The left fallopian tube (2) and round ligament (3) are lifted forwards and the ovary (4), bladder (5) and small intestine (6) are all visible.

2A View of posterior wall fibroid

The uterus is lifted forward to show a moderate-sized intramural fibroid (1) on the left posterolateral wall; it is apparently a single fibroid. The fundus of the uterus is raised on the surface of the fibroid and pushed to the right.

2B Haemostatic clamps for myomectomy

The illustration shows a Bonney's myomectomy clamp (1), rubber-covered bowel clamps for the ovarian pedicle (2), and various bulldog artery clamps which may also be used for the ovarian pedicles (3).

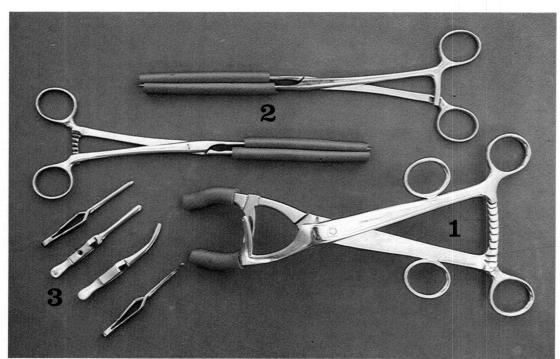

Stage 1: Application of haemostatic clamps

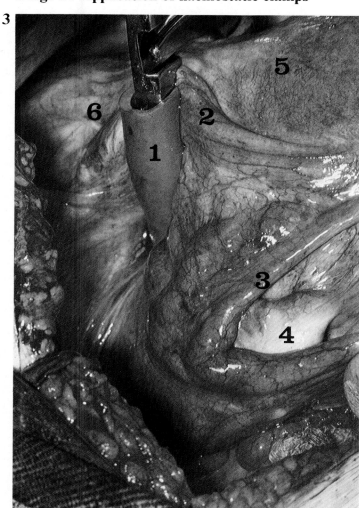

3 Application of Bonney's myomectomy clamp

It is an enormous advantage if haemostasis can be assured during myomectomy, otherwise the fibroid cavity sometimes fills up rapidly with blood and it is not possible to make an unhurried and neat obliteration of the cavity. The uterine vessels can be controlled either by the use of a Bonney's myomectomy clamp, as shown, or by making an opening in the broad ligament on each side lower down at the level of the internal cervical os, and passing a rubber tube or catheter round the uterus to act as a tourniquet. The Bonney clamp has the great advantage of supporting or fixing the uterus in the wound once it is in place. It is applied from the anterior aspect low down on to the uterus (1) and takes the inner ends of the round ligaments (2) in its grasp. The left tube (3) and the left ovary (4) are seen. The number (5) indicates the anterior aspect of the uterus and (6) the cervix.

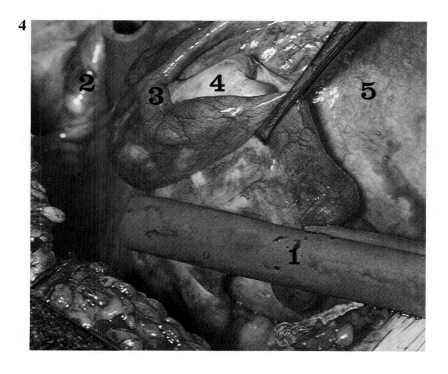

4 Haemostatic clamp on ovarian pedicle

It is not sufficient merely to control the uterine vessels and the blood supply from the ovarian arteries is controlled in this case by using a small bowel clamp (1) with the blades sheathed in rubber and one is placed on the infundibulopelvic ligament on each side. The left round ligament (2), the left tube (3), the left ovary (4) and the uterus (5) are all seen. Bowel clamps can sometimes be an embarrassment by their size in the operative field and neater alternatives are bulldog arterial clamps with the jaws sheathed in rubber. Ring forceps or sponge forceps are sometimes used but we consider them too harsh and liable to traumatise the tissues. If removal of the fibroids takes more than 20 to 25 minutes, the clamps should be temporarily released and retightened to avoid continuing anoxia.

5

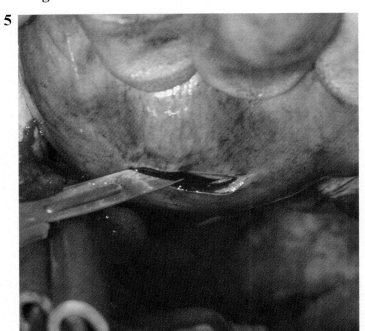

6

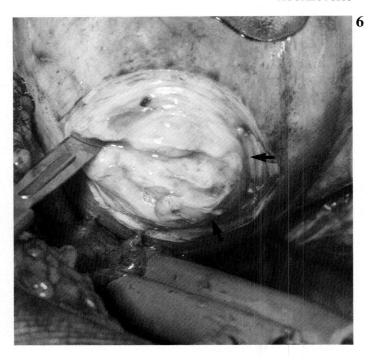

5 to 7 Incision into uterus and fibroid

An incision of the minimal length to allow removal of the fibroid is made through the uterine wall over the apex of the fibroid in Figure 5. The incision is carried quite deeply into the underlying fibroid itself as shown in Figure 6; it is of no consequence if the fibroid is partially bisected. The capsule of the fibroid is clearly visible (arrowed) and is being held back by tissue forceps (1) and (2) in Figure 7. The fibroid itself is mobilised by a Greville-MacDonald dissector (3).

7

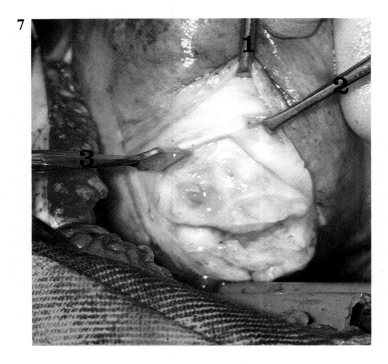

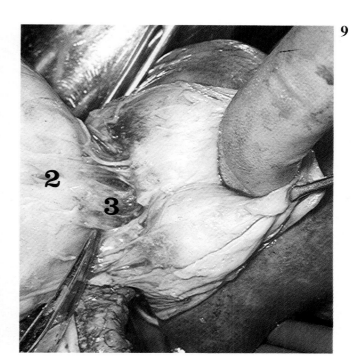

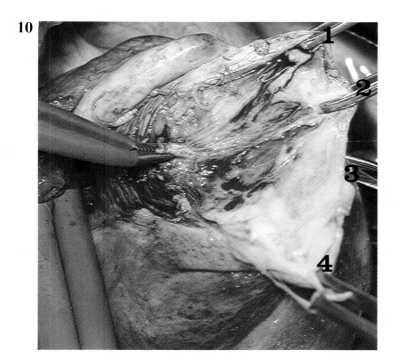

8 to 10 Enucleation of fibroid

In Figure 8 the forefinger (1) is used to supplement the dissector in freeing the fibroid from its capsule (2). Littlewood's forceps pull on the fibroid (3) and the line of separation is arrowed.

In Figure 9 the fibroid (2) is almost completely enucleated and the scissors are separating fibrous strands at (3).

In Figure 10 the fibroid has been removed and the cavity is held open by tissue forceps (1, 2, 3, 4) while the diathermy seals off a torn blood vessel in the depth of the cavity.

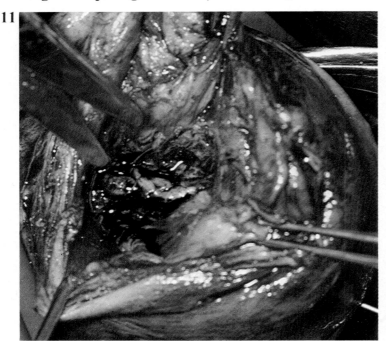

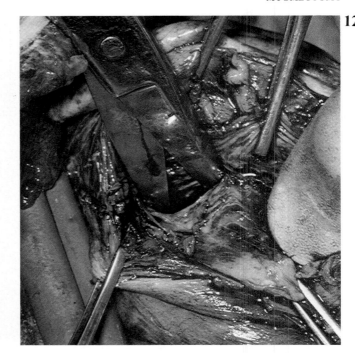

11 to 13 Opening into endometrial cavity

It is desirable to open through the fibroid cavity into the uterine cavity. This allows exploration of the uterus for fibroids obtruding into it, but the main reason is to allow drainage of blood from the fibroid cavity postoperatively. The blood drains into the uterus and out from the cervix into the vagina and this is a most important safety valve. In Figure 11 the cavity left by the enucleated fibroid is held open by tissue forceps and the scissors are about to seek the endometrial cavity in its depth. In Figure 12 the scissors have opened into the endometrial cavity and the blades are being opened. In Figure 13 the surgeon's finger explores the uterine cavity through the fibroid cavity.

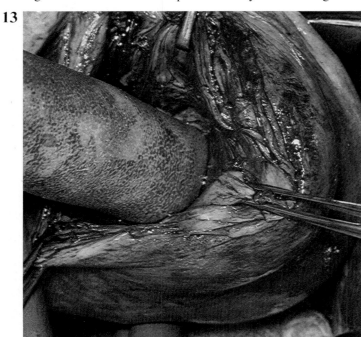

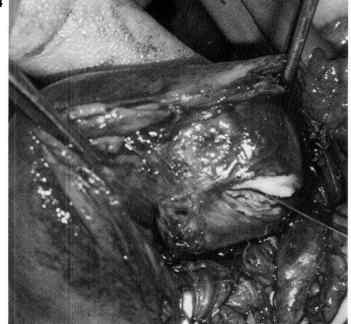

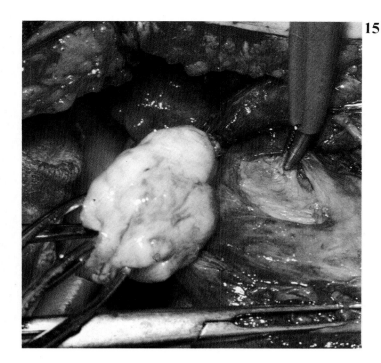

14 to 16 Removal of second fibroid through lateral tunnelling incision

The cavity of the larger fibroid is used as a stage in the enucleation of a smaller fibroid lying lateral to it. The wall of the cavity is incised over the palpable second fibroid in a lateral direction and in effect tunnelling towards it. This is shown in Figure 14. In Figure 15 the second fibroid is enucleated and held in tissue forceps while a torn or bleeding vessel is being sealed by diathermy. In Figure 16 the secondary cavity of the smaller fibroid is being closed by interrupted PGA No. 00 sutures. One suture is already in position (1) and the second is being inserted (2). The still open primary cavity is visible.

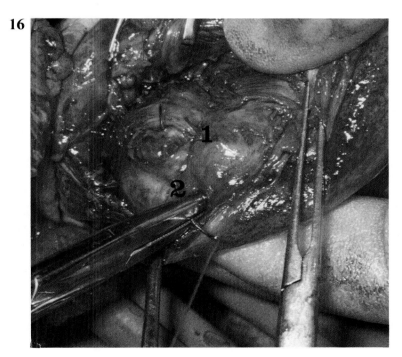

Stage 4: Closure of fibroid cavity in layers

17

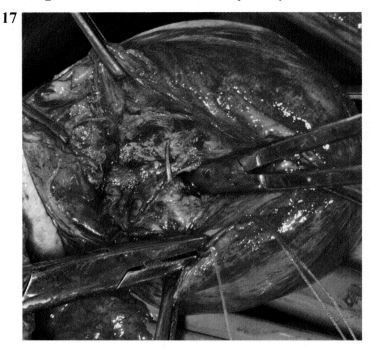

18

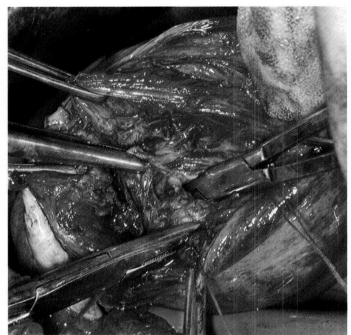

17 to 19 Closure of fibroid cavity (first layer)

The primary cavity is now closed and as it is fairly large this is done in a series of steps or layers beginning in the depth of the cavity and working towards the peritoneal surface. Figure 17 shows the needle carrying a PGA No. 0 suture pick up the first bite of uterine muscle deep in the cavity and in Figure 18 transfixing the corresponding shoulder of tissue on the other side. In Figure 19 the first stitch is being tied off. The forceps (1) shows the opening into the uterine cavity and the fibroid cavity itself is held open by tissue forceps. Two further similar sutures will close this first layer.

19

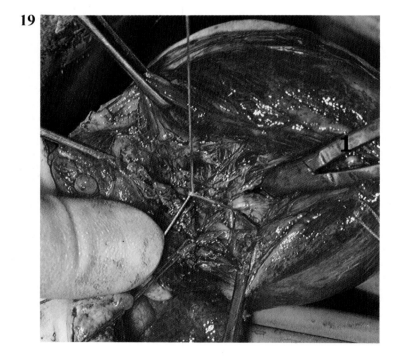

20

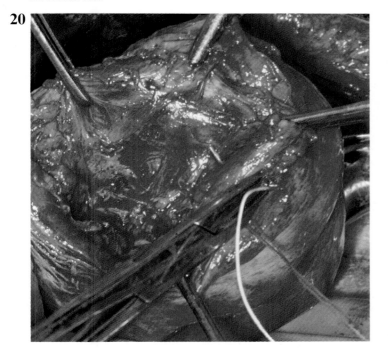

21

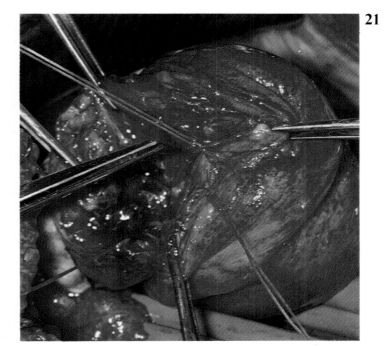

20 to 23 Closure of fibroid cavity (second layer)

The same procedure is followed at a more superficial level. The illustrations show the placement of the first stitch in Figure 20 and its completion in Figure 21. A second stitch is placed and ready to cut in Figures 22 and 23 respectively.

22

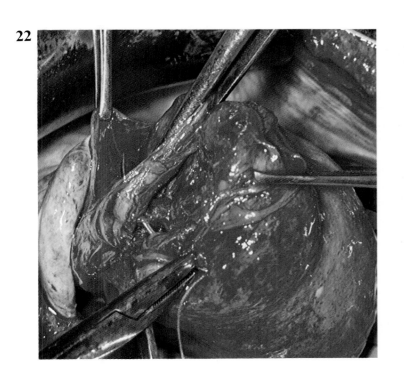

23

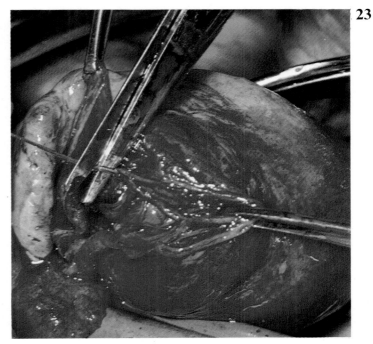

24
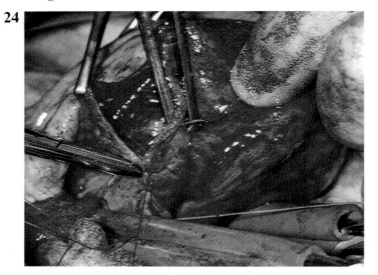

25
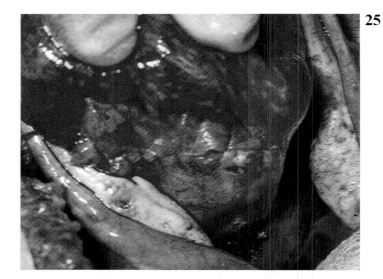

26

27
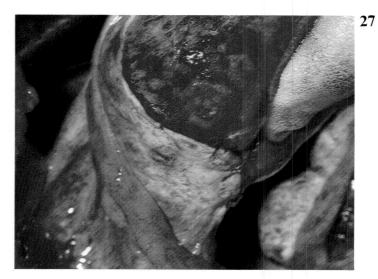

28
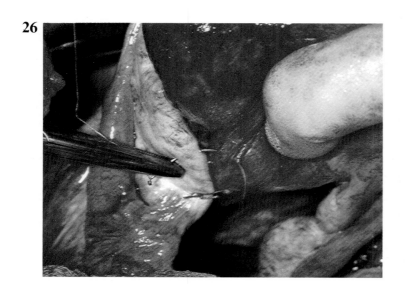

24 to 28 Closure of peritoneal surface (superficial layer)

A continuous inverting suture of PGA No. 00 has begun in Figure 24 and is proceeding along the wound. The needle pierces the wound edge from within outwards on each side in turn as shown in the photograph and this gives an inverted smooth suture line of herring-bone appearance. Figure 25 shows the cavity closed and in close proximity to a mobile left ovary. The opportunity to cover the incision by available structures is always taken and in Figure 26 this is being done. Figure 27 shows the incision covered completely; Figure 28 shows the excised fibroids.

Removal of multiple fibroids

In this case there are several fibroids and in particular one low on the anterior uterine wall close to the bladder. This gives the opportunity of showing the incision made through the uterovesical peritoneum, which in this situation is loose and thereby gives a safe coverage to the incision later. The posterior fibroid cannot be covered by loose peritoneum in this case and depends on the inverting stitch for smooth closure.

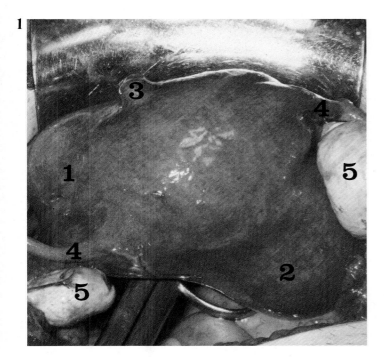

1 General view on opening the abdomen
There is a moderate-sized fibroid on the anterior wall of the uterus looking down (1) and a larger one on the upper right posterior wall (2) with a tiny subserous fibroid (3) anteriorly. The tubes (4) and ovaries (5) are visible and the uterus is supported anteriorly on the scissors. A Bonney's clamp could only have been placed posteriorly before removing the anterior fibroid and was not used in the first place.

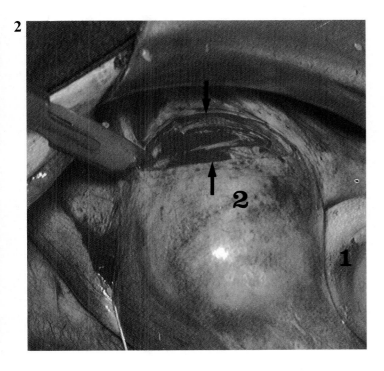

Stage 1: Opening of uterovesical pouch

2 Exposure of fibroid
An incision through the loose peritoneal fold is made transversely much as in a hysterectomy and the lower leaf falls back to expose the fibroid which is then cut into as previously described. Note the finger (1) supporting the fibroid (2) while the incision is made. The upper and lower edges of the peritoneum are arrowed.

175

Stage 2: Enucleation of fibroids and closure of cavity

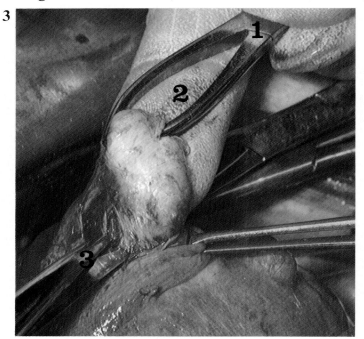

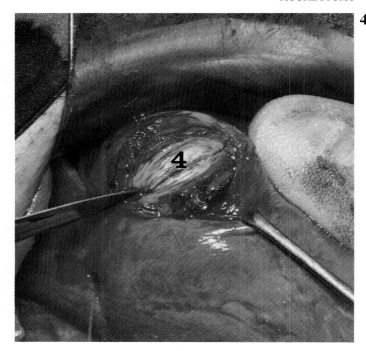

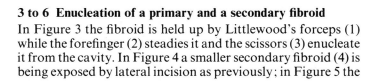

3 to 6 Enucleation of a primary and a secondary fibroid

In Figure 3 the fibroid is held up by Littlewood's forceps (1) while the forefinger (2) steadies it and the scissors (3) enucleate it from the cavity. In Figure 4 a smaller secondary fibroid (4) is being exposed by lateral incision as previously; in Figure 5 the two contiguous fibroids are being shelled out with the help of the Greville-MacDonald dissector (5). In Figure 6 the finger explores the uterine cavity which has been opened as previously described.

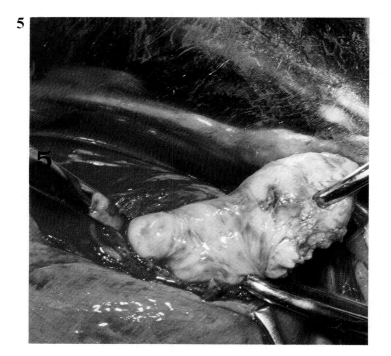

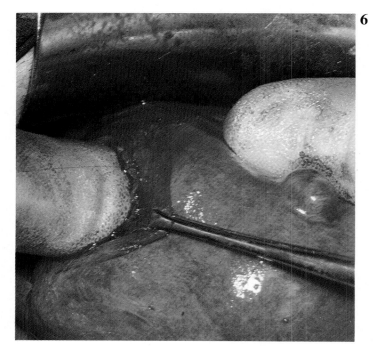

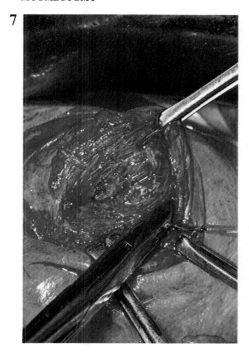

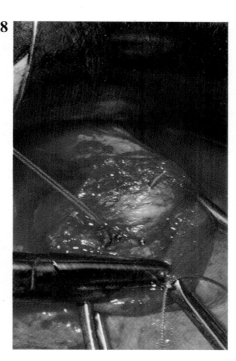

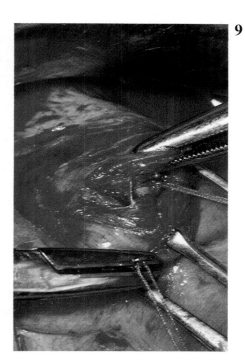

7 to 11 Closure and covering of fibroid cavity

The cavity is closed in two layers. Figure 7 shows the placement of the first stitch of the deepest layer of the cavity. Figure 8 shows the first stitch of the second layer with an uncut suture of the first layer keeping the cavity everted. A second stitch in the second layer is shown in Figure 9. Figure 10 shows the commencement of closure of the peritoneum of the uterovesical pouch; in Figure 11 the myomectomy site is covered by the closed peritoneum.

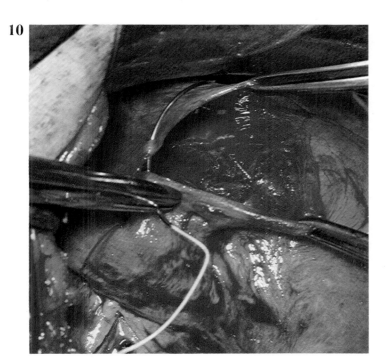

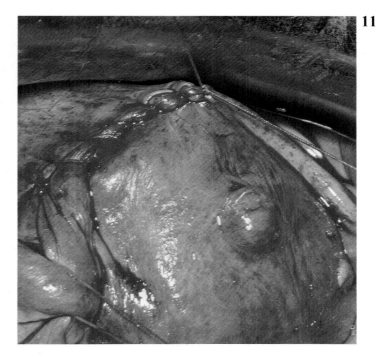

12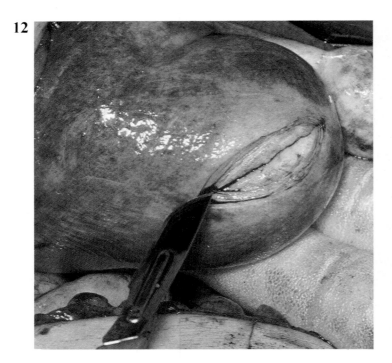

13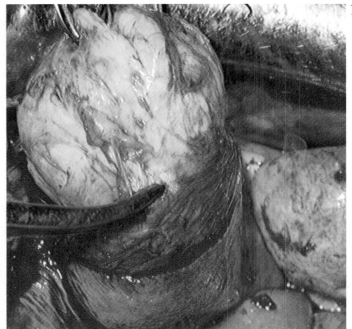

12 to 14 Enucleation of posterior-wall fibroid

The incision is made in the usual fashion in Figure 12, the fibroid is being enucleated in Figure 13 and blood vessels are clamped before its complete separation in Figure 14.

14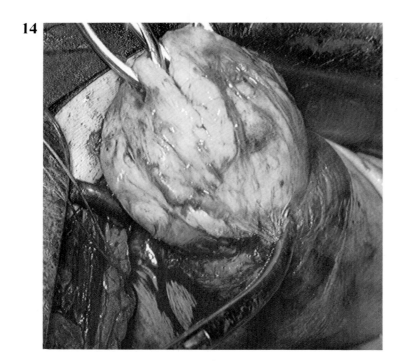

Stage 3: Opening of endometrial cavity: closure of fibroid cavity

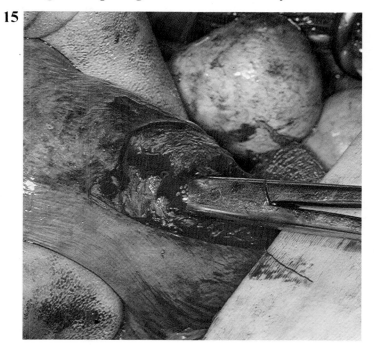

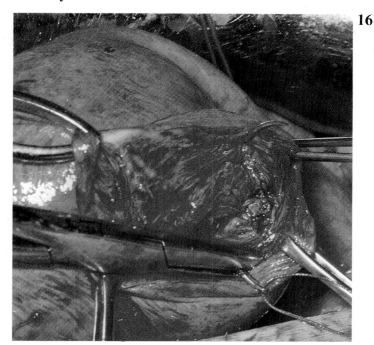

15 to 17 Opening into endometrial cavity and commencing closure of fibroid cavity

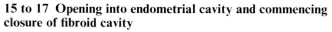

In Figure 15 continuity with the endometrial cavity is established by means of a Spencer-Wells forceps. The reasons for opening into the uterine lumen have been discussed in the previous section.

In Figure 16 the first stitch of the deepest layer is being placed. In Figure 17 the first stitch is still uncut while the second is being inserted.

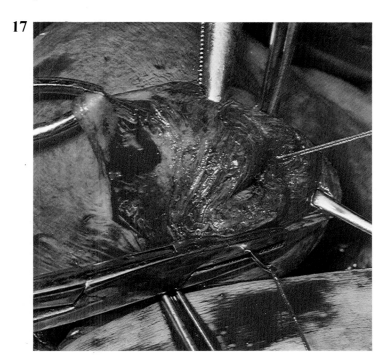

18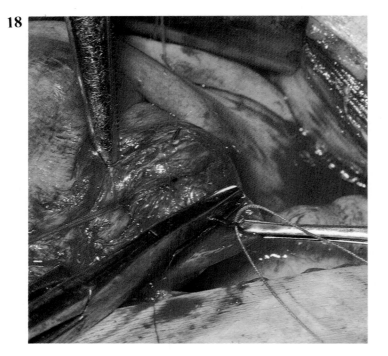

19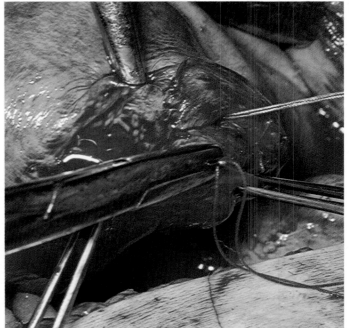

18 and 19 Closure of fibroid cavity (second layer)

In Figure 18 the first stitch of the second layer is being placed. In Figure 19 the first stitch is still uncut while the second is being inserted.

Stage 4: Peritonisation of wound area

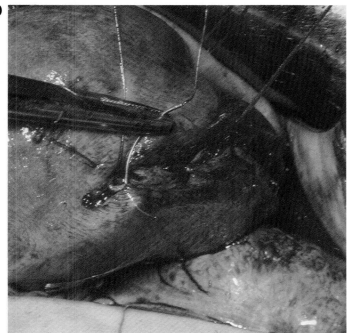

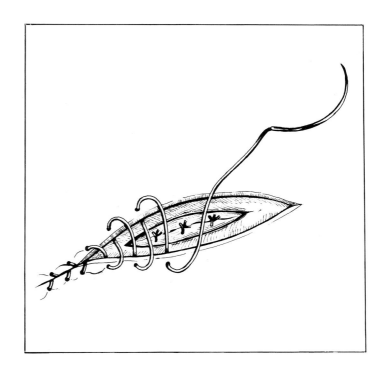

20 and 21 Superficial closure with inverting stitch

In Figure 20 an anchor stitch has been tied and the wound is being closed by an inverting suture which pierces each wound edge from within outwards as shown in the diagram. Figure 21 shows the smooth surface of the uterus which results. There is little prospect of adhesion to surrounding structures.

21

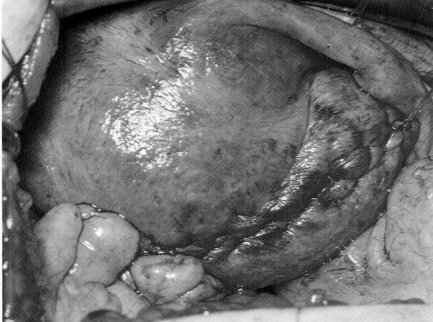

5: Tubo-ovarian surgery

Surgery of the fallopian tube when related to the treatment of infertility or extrauterine pregnancy is described in Volumes 4 and 6 of this Atlas series. Ovarian malignancy is a special problem normally requiring pelvic clearance if that is possible and is dealt with in Volume 3. Apart from these conditions, there is a large group of benign ovarian cysts of multiple type which may undergo various complications such as torsion, rupture and degeneration. Typical operations for such circumstances are described. Sterilisation by tubal ligation has become a major part of modern gynaecological practice and the procedures commonly used are described.

Ovarian cystectomy

Of the non-malignant conditions simple ovarian cysts and dermoid tumours are suitable for ovarian cystectomy; the basic technique is described below.

Such cysts vary enormously in size and although the same principles are followed in their removal, care must be taken to preserve adequate ovarian tissue where it is thinly spread out over the ovarian pole of a large cyst. In such circumstances reconstitution of the affected ovary includes forming it into a compact gonad.

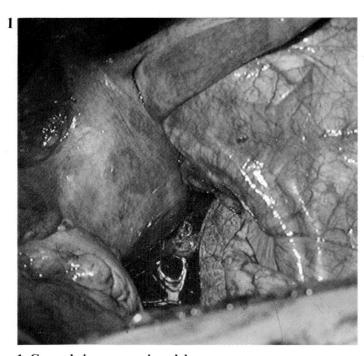

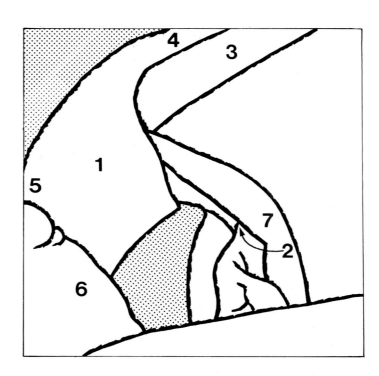

1 General view on opening abdomen
The right infundibulopelvic fold is raised on the surface of an enlarged right ovary which is not visible and the right tube is distorted and spread out over the raised area. The right round ligament is also on the stretch anteriorly. The patient is known to have a right ovarian cyst but its type is not immediately obvious. It is important to note at this stage that the left ovary is apparently normal.

1 Uterus
2 Infundibulopelvic fold with underlying ovary
3 Right fallopian tube
4 Right round ligament
5 Left round ligament
6 Left ovary
7 Right external iliac artery

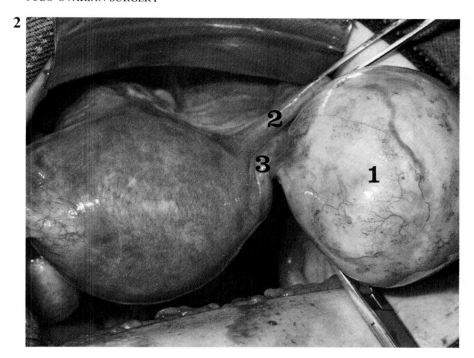

2 Cyst delivered into wound

The right ovary (1) is hooked out from under the in-fundibulopelvic ligament with the finger and is seen to be free of adhesions and with the appearance of a dermoid cyst.

The uterus is held forwards by tissue forceps attached to the right round ligament (2) and the right fallopian tube (3) is now anterior to the ovary.

Stage 1: Enucleation of cyst

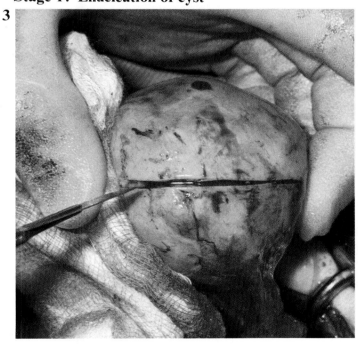

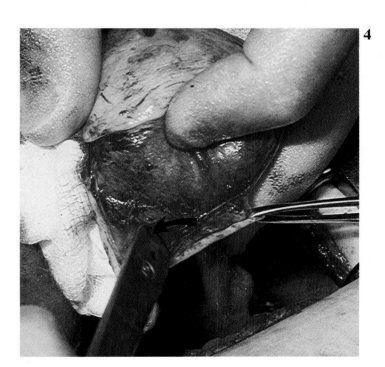

3 and 4 Enucleation of ovarian cyst (1)

In Figure 3 a transverse incision through the thickness of the ovarian capsule is made with a gentle stroke of the scalpel taking care not to injure the underlying cyst. The cut edge is held in tissue forceps in Figure 4 while the handle of the scalpel is used as a dissector to separate the cyst from its capsule. The arrow indicates the direction of this manoeuvre. The plane of separation is always easy to find.

5

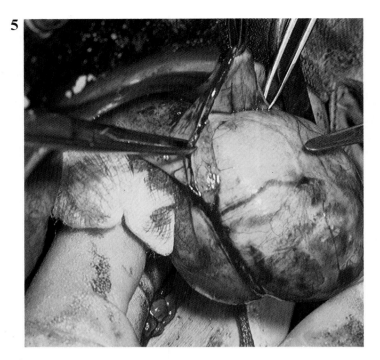

5 Enucleation of ovarian cyst (2)
The process continues until the cyst is completely enucleated and separation is aided by scissors. There is minimal bleeding.

Stage 2: Reconstruction of ovary

6

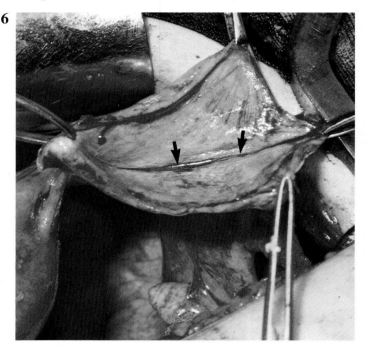

7

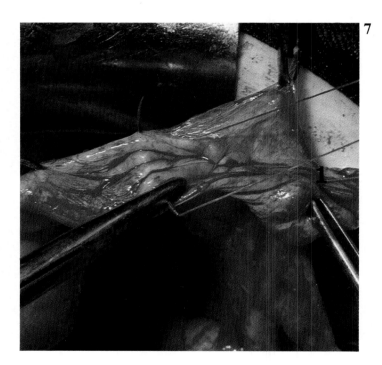

6 and 7 Reconstruction of ovary (1)
Figure 6 shows the empty capsule of the ovarian cyst held open by tissue forceps. It is thin-walled except at the hilum (arrowed) and it is necessary to reconstitute the ovary. In Figure 7 a PGA No. 00 continuous suture has been anchored at (1) and is being placed along the length of the capsule bed to close and compact the ovary. The method of inserting the stitch is shown in the following figures.

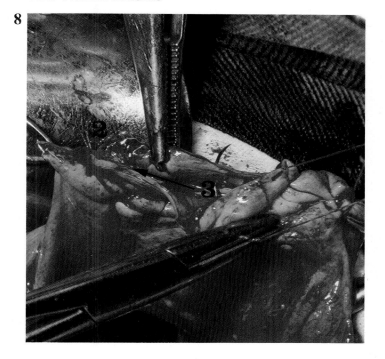

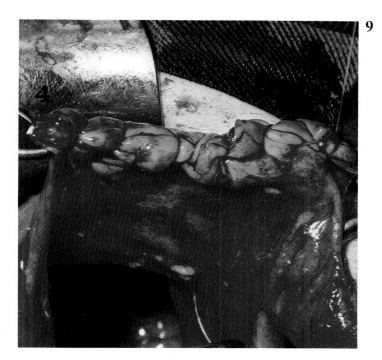

8 to 11 Reconstruction of ovary (2)

In Figure 8 the previous stitch has been completed and tied off (2) and the second over-and-over closing and haemostatic stitch (3) is being placed from right to left as arrowed. This stitch reaches the other end of the incision in Figure 9 (4) but is not tied and immediately returns back along the edge to form a continuous X stitch with itself (5) as shown in Figure 10 and from left to right as arrowed. The stitch is completed by tying to its uncut anchored end; the effect is to bunch up and shorten the ovary in addition to its haemostatic and closing function (Figure 11). This means that there is one deep suture line (Figure 7) and a double surface stitch (Figures 8 to 11).

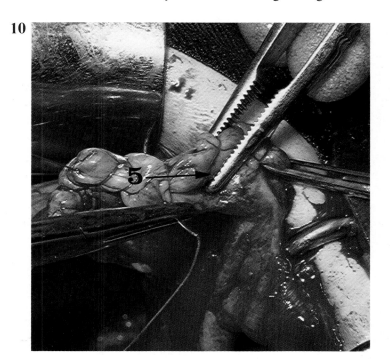

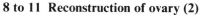

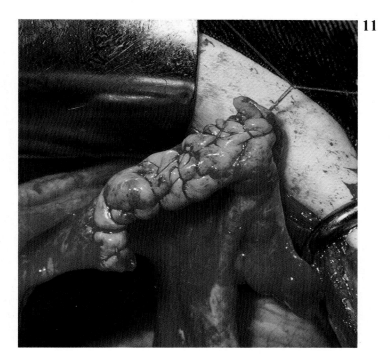

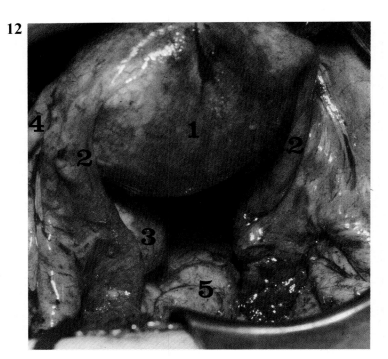

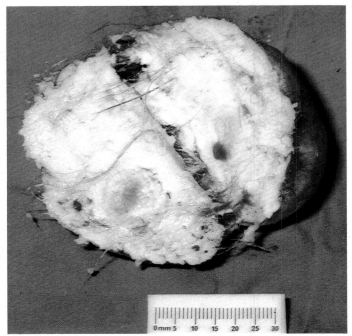

12 Appearance following ovarian cystectomy

The genital structures now have a completely normal appearance when seen from the posterior aspect. They are numbered as follows: (1) uterus, (2) fallopian tubes, (3) left ovary; right ovary hidden by right tube, (4) left round ligament and (5) rectum.

13 Specimen

The cut specimen is a typical benign teratoma of semi-solid consistency. Because there is a propensity for such tumours to be bilateral, the other ovary was examined carefully but no evidence of a cyst was found. Some feel that the other ovary should be split open for examination in such circumstances, but such a step we feel is not generally justified.

Salpingo-oophorectomy

Salpingo-oophorectomy or ovariotomy is much more frequently required than ovarian cystectomy and standard procedures are described. The size of the ovarian mass and the degree of involvement with surrounding structures varies enormously, so that changes in technique are sometimes essential. To cover possible eventualities a series of cases illustrating particular problems are described.

A benign cyst undergoing torsion

A benign cyst undergoing torsion is taken as a case to illustrate the standard procedure. Although not concerned with specific indications for operations in the Atlas, it should be pointed out that torsion of the appendages without necrosis does not necessarily require salpingo-oophorectomy. A cystectomy can be done and the appendages are fixed in position so that torsion does not recur.

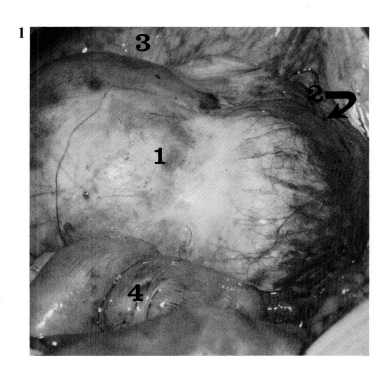

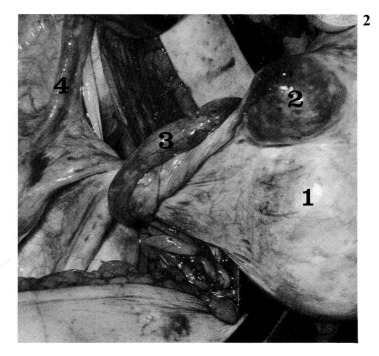

1 General view on opening abdomen
A large cyst (1) is arising from the pelvis with its pedicle hidden on the right side in the general area (2). The bladder (3) is obvious anteriorly and the bowel (4) proximal to the cyst.

2 Right ovarian cyst undergoing torsion
The cystic ovary (1) with a corpus luteum (2) has twisted in a clockwise direction through one and a half turns and the right tube (3) is incorporated in the twisted pedicle. The right round ligament is also visible (4). There is a certain amount of congestion of the appendages but there is no evidence of necrosis.

3

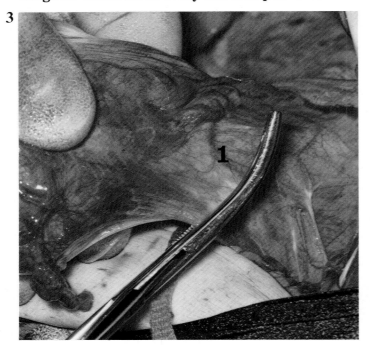

4

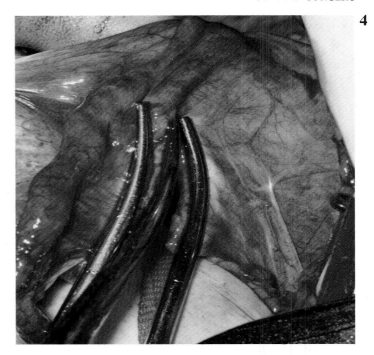

3 to 6 Removal of right ovary and fallopian tube

The pedicle is untwisted to give better and safer access to the vessels. In Figure 3 the ovary is held medially while the infundibulopelvic ligament (1) which contains the ovarian vessels and attached ovarian ligament is displayed. In Figure 4 it is double clamped and being divided; in Figure 5 the right broad ligament (3) and the right tube (4) are displayed for clamping. In Figure 6 the tube and ovary are being detached. Note that a good cuff of tissue is left distal to the forceps and that the pedicles are not too bulky for safe ligation. The right round ligament (5) helps to orientate the picture in Figures 5 and 6.

5

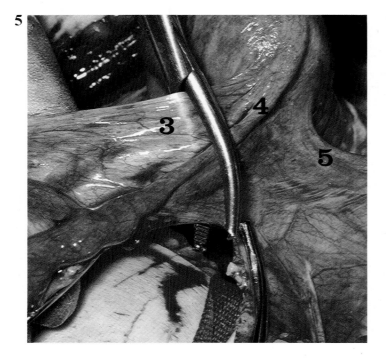

6

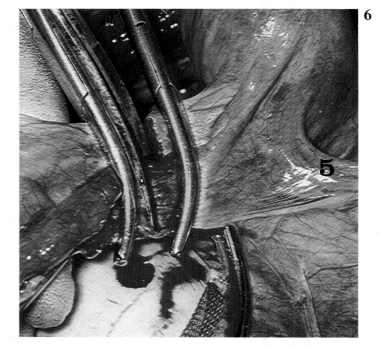

Stage 2: Transfixion and ligation of pedicles

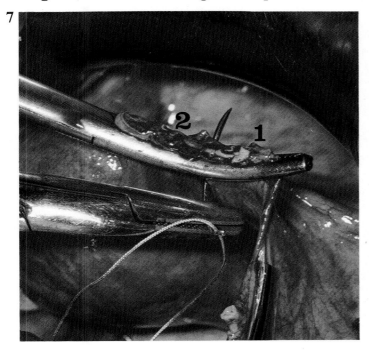

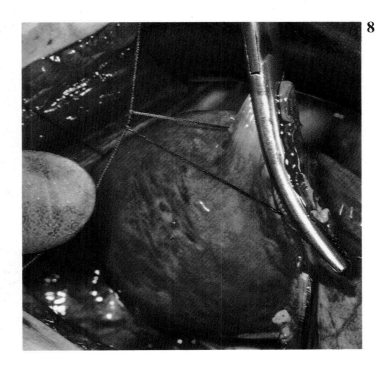

7 to 10 Securing pedicles

The bulky pedicles are transfixed, tied and double tied in the usual fashion. Figure 7 shows the medial part of the right broad ligament containing fallopian tube (2) and vessels (1) being transfixed and in Figure 8 it is tied off with PGA No. 1 suture. In Figure 9 the ovarian pedicle is transfixed and is seen to contain a large vein. In Figure 10 ligation is being completed and the previously tied pedicle is seen.

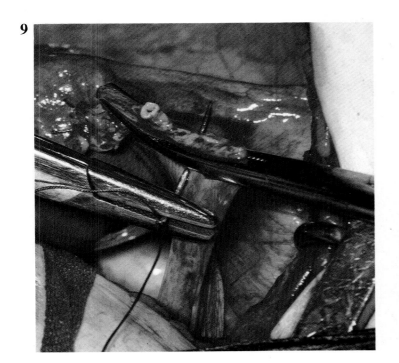

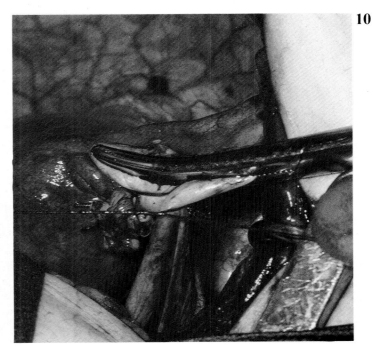

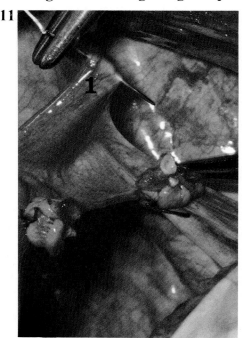
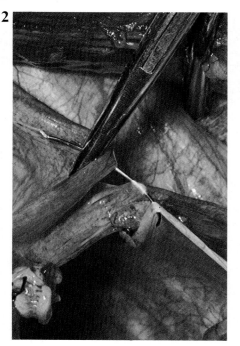
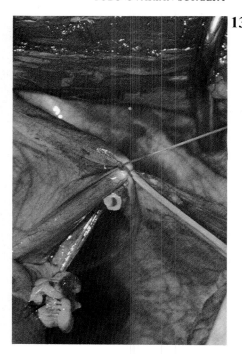

11 to 15 Covering ligated pedicles with round ligament

The neatest and most satisfactory method of covering the pedicles is to fold back the round ligament (1) over them in the manner illustrated. It carries a sheet of peritoneum with it which makes a smooth surface. In Figures 11 and 12 the lateral part of the round ligament is stitched backwards to cover the ovarian pedicle which is buried when the stitch is tied in Figure 13. In Figure 14 the stitch continues medially to fix the round ligament (1) to the posterior aspect of the broad ligament and is seen picking up the ovarian ligament (2) to cover the (medial) broad ligament pedicle (3). The stitch is tied off in Figure 15.

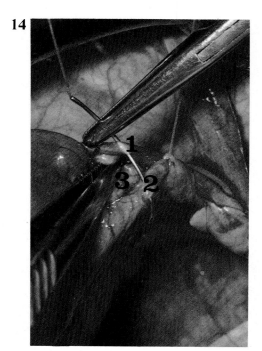
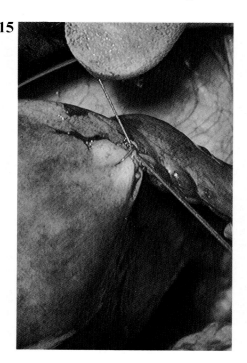
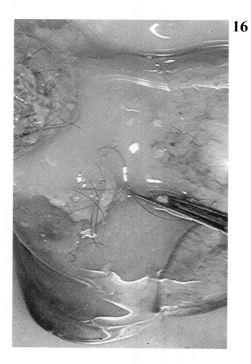

16 Specimen being opened

The cyst is seen to be a benign teratoma of semi-solid consistency. Examination of the other ovary in this case revealed a small dermoid which was shelled out and the ovary conserved.

Large mobile serous cyst

The case described here is that of a large mobile ovarian cyst, probably but not certainly benign, in a woman of 38 years of age. On the basis of the history and clinical findings the cyst was considered to be benign; the ultrasonic scan showed that the cyst was thin-walled and with no apparent solid areas. It was proposed to remove it intact and make a careful clinical and a frozen section histological examination to exclude malignancy. Apart from showing how to deal with a large cyst, the case emphasises the importance of ultra caution in dealing with ovarian cysts and tumours.

1 Negative of ultrasonic scan
The longitudinal cut of a B-scan (ultrasonic) from a diasonograph 4102 shows the outline of the cyst (1) and bladder (2). The perpendicular arrow marks the symphysis pubis.

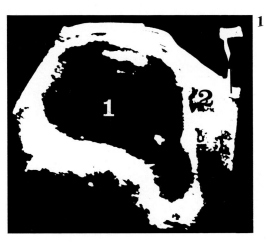

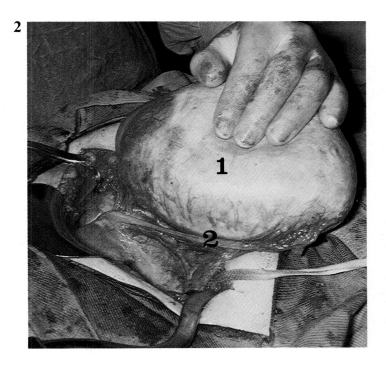

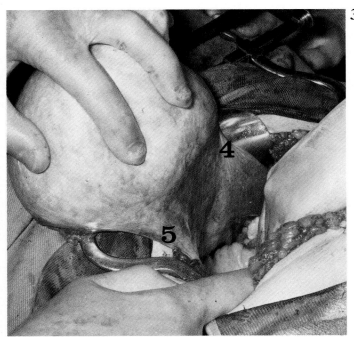

2 and 3 Appearance of ovarian cyst in wound
Figure 2 shows an anterolateral view of the left-sided cyst (1) with the left tube (2) stretched alongside and partially underneath it. The cyst is burrowing under the broad ligament and expanding forwards. In Figure 3 a posterolateral view shows a very broad pedicle from the uterine cornu (4) to the fold of the infundibulopelvic ligament (5).

4

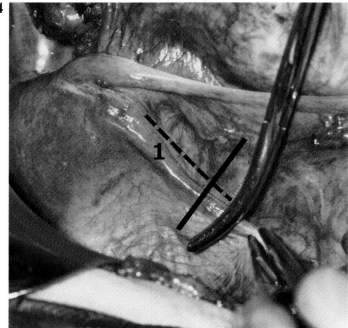

5

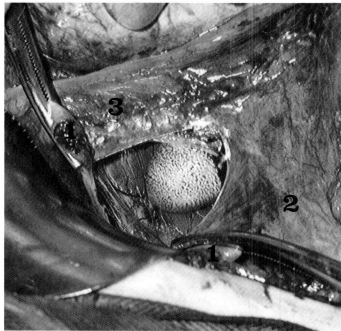

4 and 5 Mobilisation of cyst

The usual procedure is to divide the anterior layer of the broad ligament just posterior to the round ligament in the direction of the interrupted line, but in this particular instance the cyst was burrowing deeply underneath the broad ligament, putting the round ligament on the stretch and obliterating the broad ligament space. It was considered safer to divide the round ligament along the continuous line at right angles to the other

and dividing the round ligament itself to obtain improved access. The round ligament is displayed (1) in Figure 4 and has been divided between forceps in Figure 5. The finger is now visible at the back of the broad ligament and shows the pedicle of the cyst split into its two attachments, one is the infundibulopelvic pedicle (2) and the other is the attachment to the uterus (3). Each pedicle will now be doubly clamped and cut between the forceps to free the cyst and accompanying tube.

6

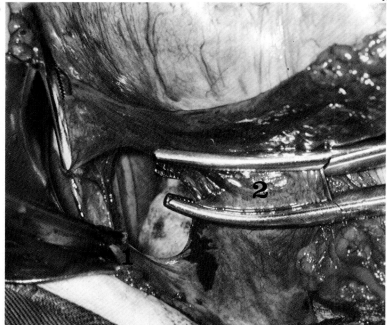

7

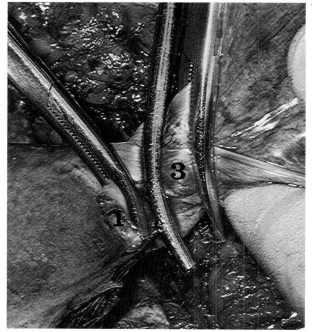

6 and 7 Removal of cyst

In Figure 6 the infundibulopelvic portion of the cyst pedicle (2) is doubly clamped and awaits division between the forceps; in Figure 7 the pedicle attached to the uterus (3) and which is made up of broad ligament, fallopian tube and ovarian

ligament is similarly clamped and ready for separation. Both ends of the cut round ligament are seen, the lateral end in Figure 6 (1) and the medial end in Figure 7 (1).

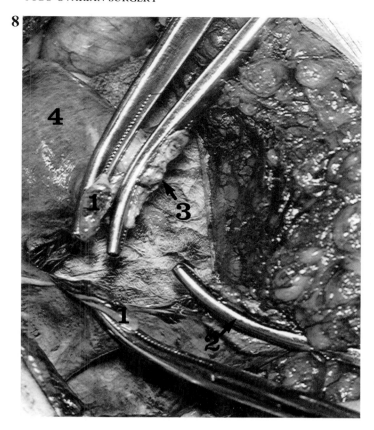

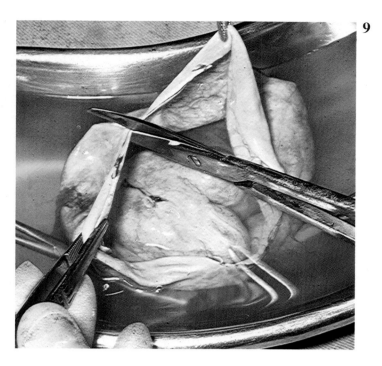

8 Appearance with cyst removed

The fundus of the uterus is numbered (4) and the various pedicles held by the forceps are as follows: (1) and (1) round ligament, (2) infundibulopelvic ligament, (3) broad ligament at uterine cornu which contains the ovarian ligament and the fallopian tube. The lumen of the latter is arrowed.

9 Opening ovarian cyst at operation

Before proceeding further with the operation the surgeon splits open the ovarian cyst with scalpel and scissors to display a smooth-walled cavity and clear cyst fluid. The ovarian tissue in the base of the cyst appears benign and there seems little risk of its being otherwise. If facilities are available as in this case frozen section histology is used to conclusively exclude malignancy.

10
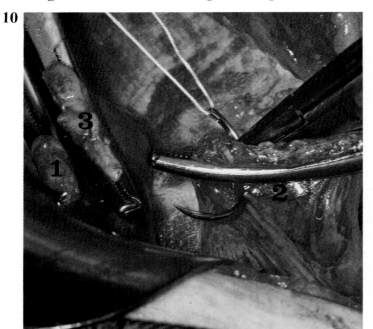

11
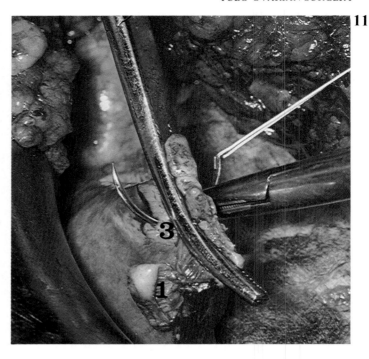

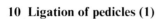

10 Ligation of pedicles (1)

The infundibulopelvic portion of the cyst pedicle (2) is being transfixed by a round-bodied needle carrying a PGA No. 1 suture and will be doubly ligated. Immediately anterior to it is the other half of the pedicle from the uterus (3) and anterior to that the uterine end of the cut round ligament (1).

11 Ligation of pedicles (2)

The uterine end of the broad ligament portion of the cyst pedicle (3) is being transfixed and will be tied in similar fashion. The uterine end of the cut round ligament has already been ligated at (1).

Stage 3: Covering of ligated pedicles

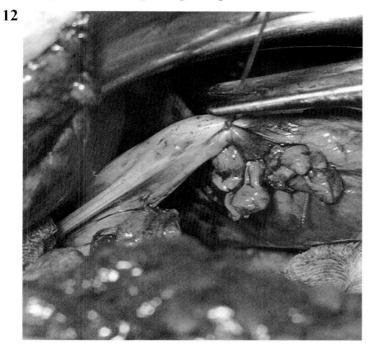

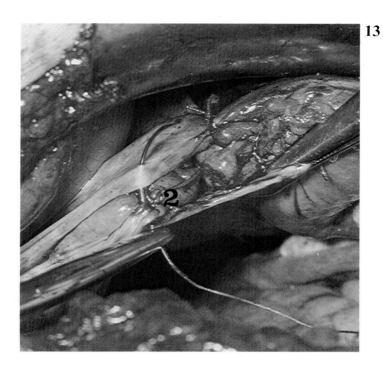

12 to 15 Covering pedicles with round ligament

The same procedure as previously is used to cover the pedicles with peritoneum. In Figure 12 the left round ligament has been reconstituted and is available to stitch to the posterior layer of the broad ligament from left to right as shown. In Figure 13 the first stitch when tied will bury the infundibulo-pelvic part of the cyst pedicle (2); this has been done in Figure 14 and the uterine part (3) is being similarly dealt with; in Figure 15 the area is completely covered.

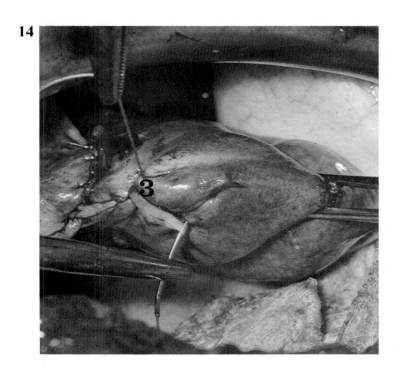

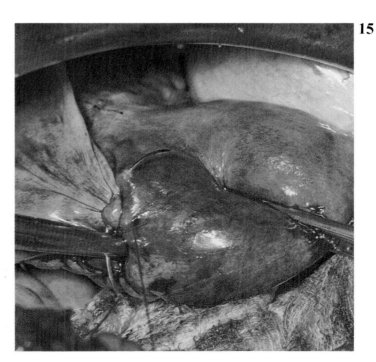

Large adherent pseudobroad ligament cyst

This large adherent pseudobroad ligament cyst developed in the left ovary of a previously hysterectomised patient and developed over a considerable length of time. The case shows possible dangers to the ureter in the removal of such a cyst and indicates how these dangers can be avoided. Symptoms were entirely related to the size of the swelling; ultrasonic scanning showed the cyst to be full of fluid and there was no indication that it was other than benign. As will be seen the cyst burrowed under the remainder of the broad ligament pushing the round ligament remnants upwards and forwards and became firmly attached to the pelvic floor extraperitoneally. Such cysts are sometimes described as pseudobroad ligament cysts. They are entirely ovarian in origin but burrow under the broad ligament like those of that name.

The cyst in this case was tapped before removal and critical comment on that will be expected. To avoid spill of malignant cells, and because it is never possible to be completely certain that a cyst is benign, teachers and textbooks advise that every cyst should be removed intact, no matter how large, no matter if the incision stretches from xiphisternum to pubis. The advice is well intentioned and good, but there are many cases with little or no likelihood of malignancy and we do not think it need be observed in every case. The authors' views on tapping very large and probably malignant cysts will be dealt with in Volume 3; large clinically benign cysts such as here are a different matter altogether. A cyst which is simply large and without adhesions can generally be removed intact through a moderately sized transverse incision and that is probably correct, although its rupture during delivery through the abdominal wound is rather inelegant and if delivered intact it must not be allowed to drag on and possibly tear the pedicle. If the cyst is adherent or has taken up an abnormal position as in this case, it becomes highly dangerous to work blindly around it. If it does remain intact access to the pedicle will be difficult. Much handling is entailed and danger to the ureter and surrounding structures is very real. If the cyst ruptures when partially separated the dangers of expressing possible tumour cells into the circulation are added to those of spill. There is much to be said for definitively tapping the cyst by a method that, for all practical purposes, eliminates spill and then proceed to an easy, controlled and safe enucleation of the contracted and thick wall of the almost empty cyst. It should not be assumed that a very long abdominal incision is without its problems. Reactionary bleeding is not uncommon. One sees weak scars or actual herniation from time to time. Limited postoperative activity and mobilisation bring its own particular problems.

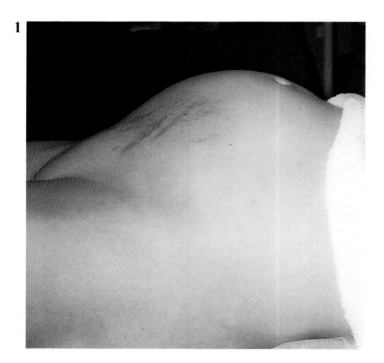

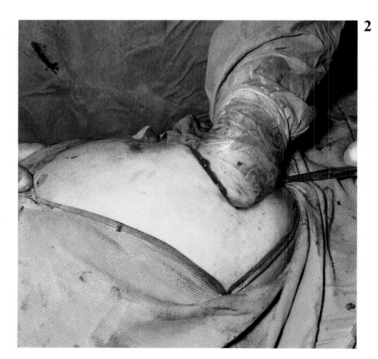

1 Abdominal swelling preoperatively
The size of the cyst can be judged from this lateral view of the abdomen which is of about 24 weeks gestation size. Note the striae on the lower abdomen.

2 Exploration of abdomen
The authors believe that exploration of the whole abdomen is a necessary preliminary to any gynaecological operation and is essential here. Adhesion of the cyst to the floor of the pelvis was confirmed and there was no question of being able to deliver the cyst into the abdominal wound.

Stage 1: Tapping and decompression of cyst

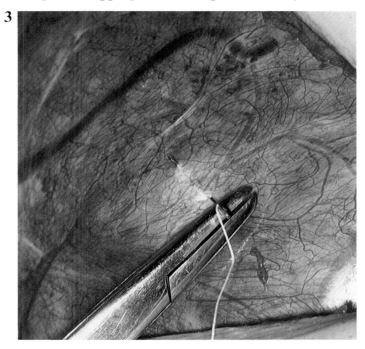

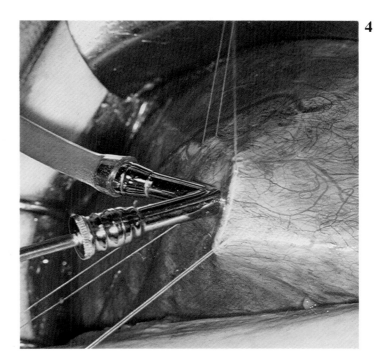

3 to 6 Tapping the cyst

The steps in the procedure are self-evident. In Figure 3 the first of a series of stay sutures is being placed using a fine needle to minimise any leakage of contents. In Figure 4 a suction trochar and cannula has been inserted and already there are signs of the cyst being decompressed. In Figure 5 the cyst is largely empty and with the cannula withdrawn the opening is clamped across by a stout forceps. A total of approximately 3,000 ml of clear fluid was removed (Figure 6).

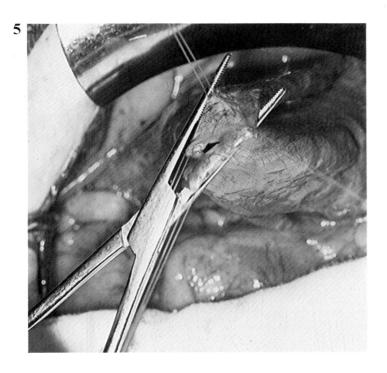

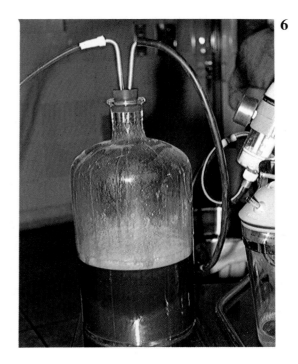

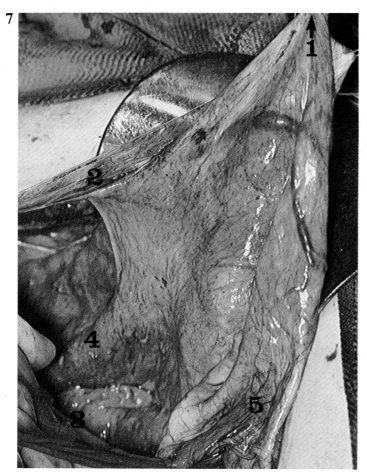

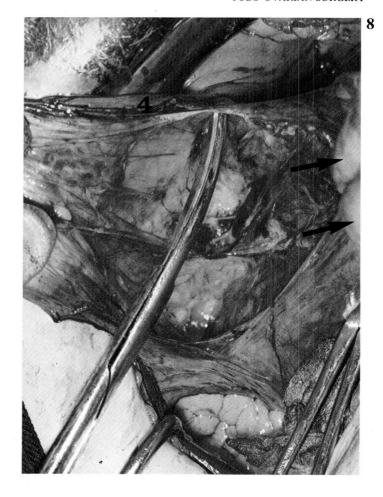

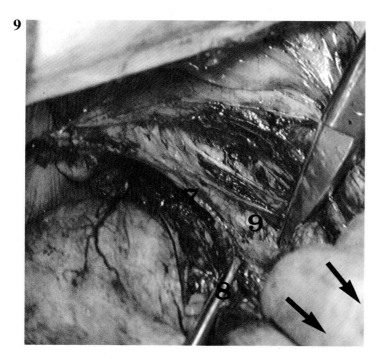

7 to 9 Reflecting peritoneum from cyst

In Figure 7 the lax empty cyst is held up by forceps at (1) and fine adhesions are seen at (2) and (3). It is lifted easily into the wound and despite the absence of landmarks removed by the previous hysterectomy the outline of the left round ligament (4) and the area of the left infundibulopelvic ligament (5) are seen. In Figure 8 the cyst is held medially in the direction of the arrows while it is freed from the anterior and left peritoneal edges held in the fingers and from the remains of the left round ligament anteriorly (4). In Figure 9 the cyst is held medially and posteriorly in the direction of the arrows and the posterior layer of peritoneum (7) is stripped downwards and is held by tissue forceps which mark the infundibulopelvic fold (8). Note the presence of the left ureter in the depth of the wound (9).

Stage 3: Definition of ureter

10

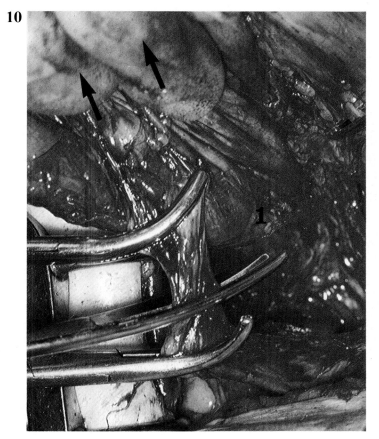

11

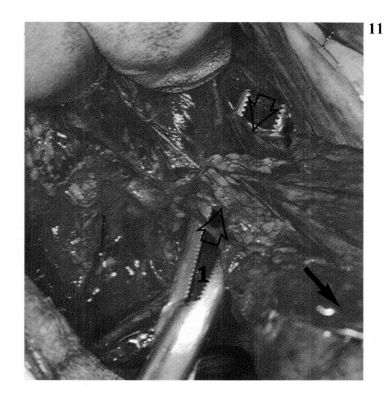

12

10 Clamping and cutting left ovarian pedicle

With the cyst held forward as arrowed the ovarian pedicle is easily identified and is dealt with as shown. The ureter is still visible at (1).

11 and 12 Defining ureter under pelvic attachment of ovarian cyst

In Figure 11 the cyst is drawn medially again (as arrowed) putting on the stretch the attachments to the pelvic floor which overlie and endanger the left ureter (1). The forceps define a tunnel (arrows define the roof); in Figure 12 the roof of this tunnel has been doubly tied and when cut between the ligatures the cyst will be released medially.

13

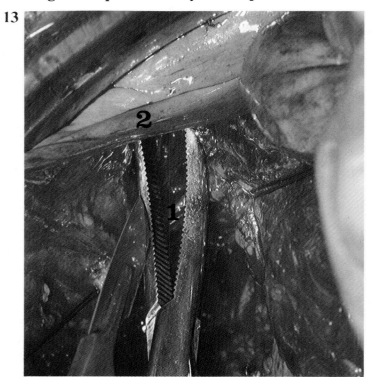

14

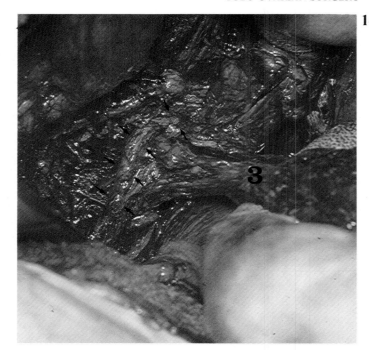

13 to 15 Separating cyst from pelvic floor

In Figure 13 the bridge of tissue over the ureter has been divided and the cyst is safely drawn medially to continue its separation. The ureter (1) is clearly seen between the blades of the forceps and the left round ligament is now obvious anteriorly (2). In Figure 14 the ureter is now clearly exposed (outlined) and a further attachment of the cyst to the pelvic floor is seen (3). This is clamped and is being divided in Figure 15. With that done the whole cyst is detached and removed from the abdomen.

15

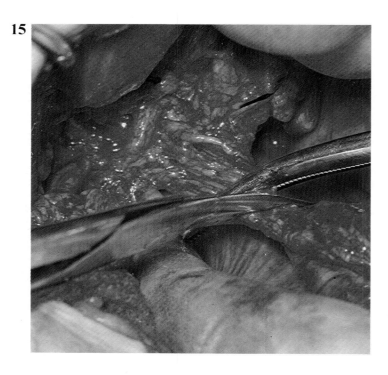

Stage 5: Peritonisation of raw area

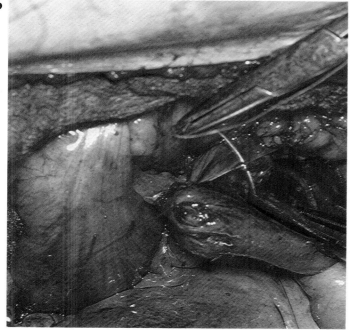

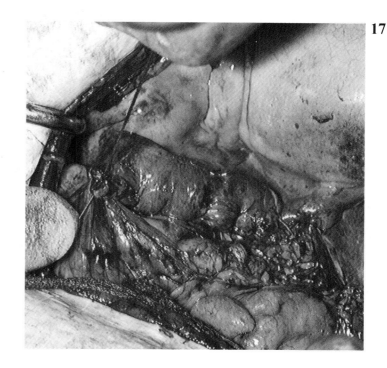

16 and 17 Closure of pelvic peritoneum

The peritoneum on the left side of the pelvis is now being approximated to cover the raw area. The first steps are being taken in Figure 16; in Figure 17 the suture is being tied off and shows an intact pelvic floor.

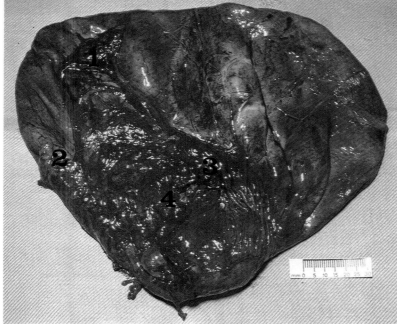

18 Specimen

The lax and now thick-walled cyst is seen to have fine adhesions at various points (1) and (2). In the general raw inferior aspect it was firmly adherent to the pelvic floor and had to be definitively separated at the two points (3) and (4).

Tubal ligation

Tubal ligation for sterilisation may be performed by a variety of methods. This is a field in which gynaecologists tend to be individualists and use a method which they have themselves evolved and which has stood them in good stead. Such methods are all modifications of the standard procedures. It is proposed in the Atlas to describe only the Pomeroy and the Irving techniques and add a note on the mini-laparotomy methods. The authors strongly advise preliminary curettage in all sterilisation operations if certain embarrassment is to be avoided sooner or later.

In some clinics it is routine practice to send the excised portions of the tubes for histological section; the report is then filed with the patient's case records. These operations are frequently performed by relatively inexperienced junior staff and the round ligament can sometimes look exactly like the medial portion of the tube and be mistaken for it. The patient on whom the operation fails may feel that her disappointment deserves some financial recompense and go to law. As a useful monitor in the first instance and as a prudent safeguard in the second, we think it advisable to have the excised tubal tissue examined and the report filed.

Pomeroy method

This simple procedure is the commonest method in current use. There is undoubtedly a small failure rate (in the region of one per cent) which may not be acceptable when strictly medical indications demand a more certain method and that will be considered later. The basic principle of the operation is to pick up a loop of the tube about its midpoint and the base of

the loop is tied with absorbable material (usually No. 1 or No. 2 plain catgut). The end or apex of the loop is excised and when the stitch absorbs the closed ends of the tube fall apart and continuity is lost. The most likely cause of failure is sinus formation where the proximal end of the tube was ligated.

Stage 1: Ligation of tube

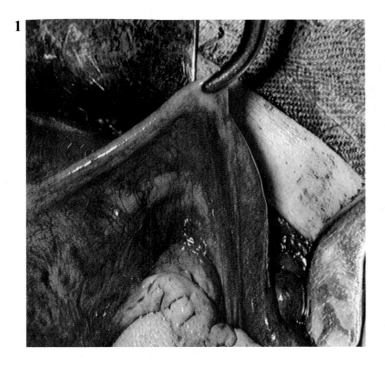

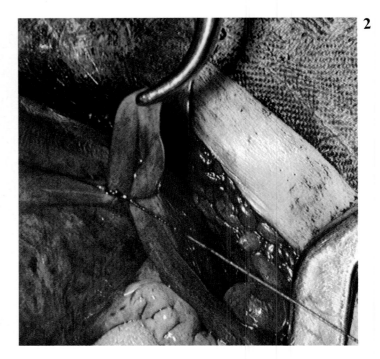

1 Definition of right fallopian tube
The right tube is picked up in forceps to form a loop in the manner shown. Some surgeons crush the base before ligating it, but that is not part of the method and is probably unwise.

2 Ligation of right tube
The base of the loop is tied firmly with No. 1 or No. 2 plain catgut as shown.

Stage 2: Excision of tube

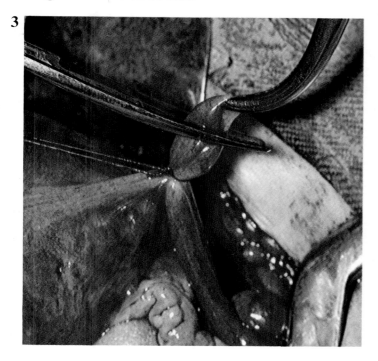

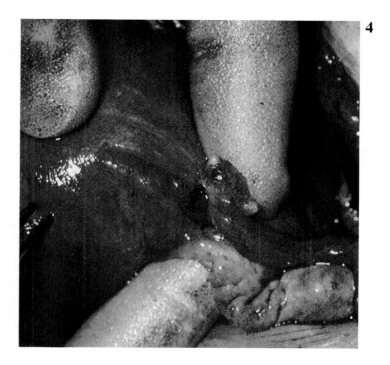

3 Excision of apex of loop
The apex of the loop is excised with scissors as shown and leaves a good cuff of tissue beyond the ligature.

4 Appearance on completion
The cut ends of the tube are clearly seen in the tied pedicle and are already at least 1 cm apart. The aim is that they will fall further apart as the ligature absorbs.

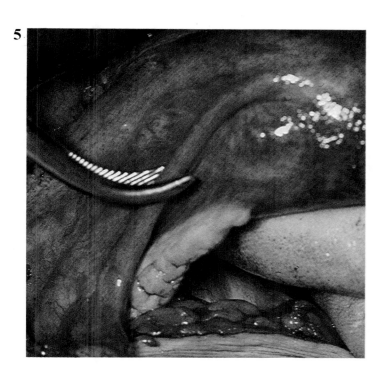

5 Definition of left tube
A loop is about to be pulled up as on the other side.

6
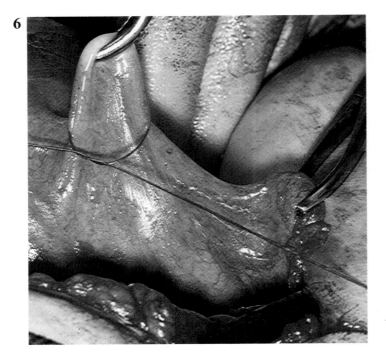

7

6 Ligation of left tube
As on right side.

7 Excision of apex of loop
As on right side.

8
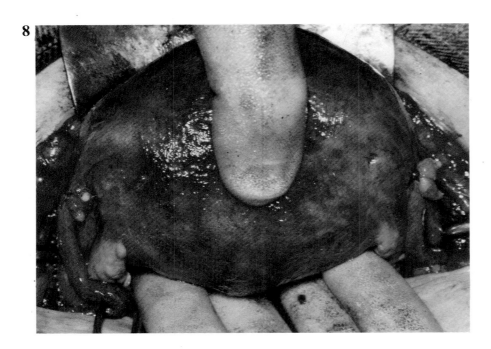

8 Appearance at completion of operation
There is no bleeding and the sites of ligature can be seen clearly. No attempt is made to cover the divided ends of the tubes.

Irving method

The Irving method is considered the most reliable of all and should be the method of choice when certainty of result is very important. It is an easy operation which takes only a few minutes to complete. The diagrams I and II show the principles of the operation. The tube is divided (1) and its medial end (2) is implanted in a tunnel (3) in the wall of the uterus. This method ought to be foolproof. In the very few occasions it has failed, it must be suspected that the surgeon's technique was faulty.

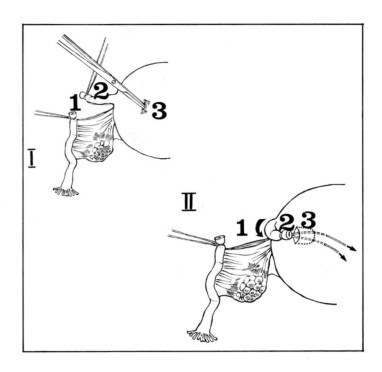

Stage 1: Definition, dissection and division of tube

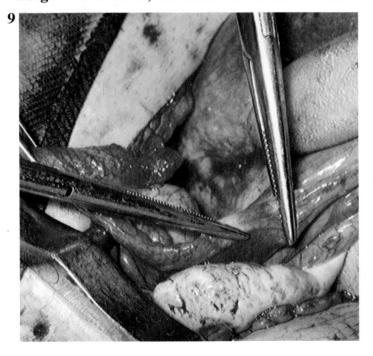

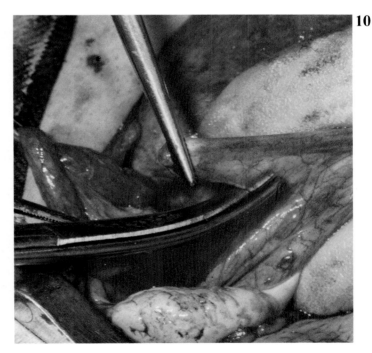

9 Definition and division of left fallopian tube

The tube is picked up by two pairs of fine artery forceps about its midpoint and is then divided with scissors. A piece of tube is excised for histological examination as recommended above.

10 Dissecting medial part of divided tube

The mesosalpinx is carefully dissected to avoid blood vessels and define and free a 2 cm length of the medial part of the divided tube.

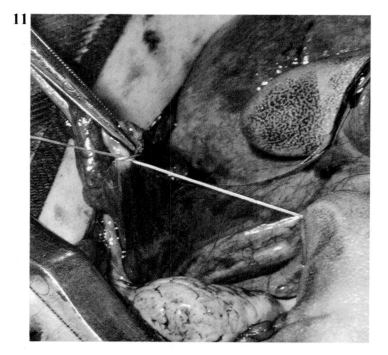

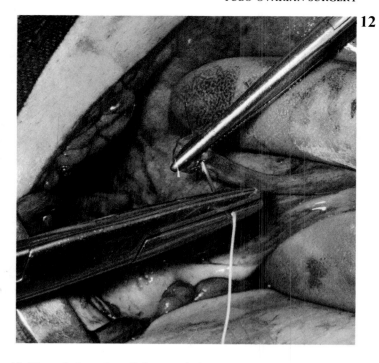

11 Ligation of lateral part of divided tube
The cut end of the lateral half of the tube is tied with PGA No. 00 or similar absorbable suture which is cut short.

12 Transfixion of medial part of divided tube
The end of this part of the tube is transfixed with a PGA No. 00 suture as shown.

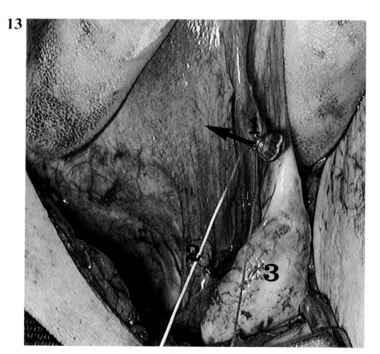

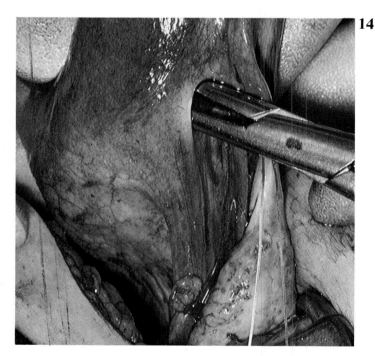

13 Appearance of prepared medial part of tube
The ligated medial part of the tube (1) with uncut suture is ready to be implanted into the uterine wall. The ligated lateral half is seen (2) and the ovary is numbered (3). The site of implantation of the tube into the uterine wall is arrowed. It should be chosen so that the tube will enter without undue stretching and at the same time will avoid the uterine vessels in the coronal plane of the uterus.

14 Forming tunnel in uterine wall
With fine-pointed Rankin-Kelly or similar forceps an oblique tunnel is made in the uterine wall as shown and the blades of the forceps opened to give access to the suture carrying needle.

Stage 2: Implantation of tube in uterine wall

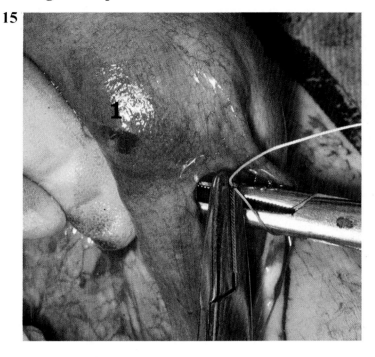

15

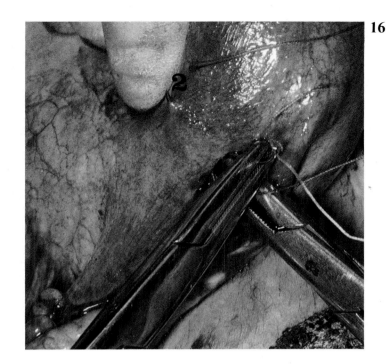

16

15 to 18 Implanting medial part of tube in uterine wall

In Figure 15 one end of the suture enters the tunnel and emerges through the muscle wall (1). In Figure 16 the process is repeated with the other end of the stitch (2). In Figure 17 they are drawn tight ready for tying and in Figure 18 have been tied off to hold the tube within the tunnel.

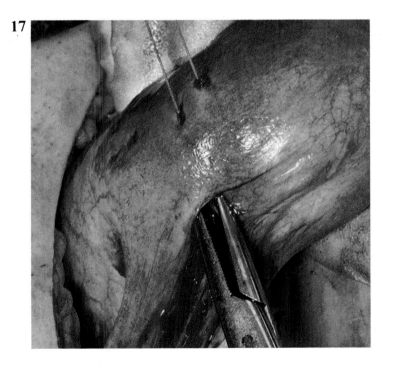

17

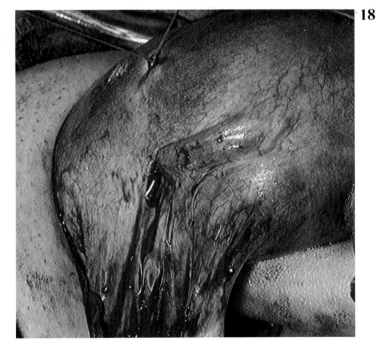

18

19

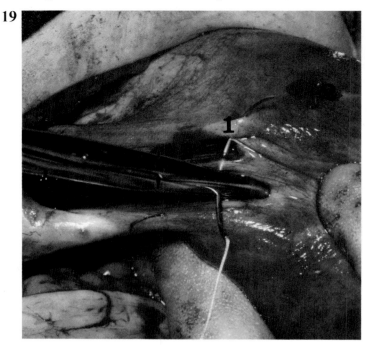

20

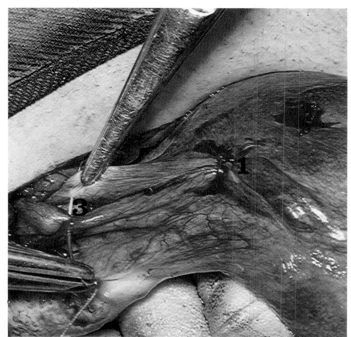

19 to 21 Closure of peritoneum over site of implantation and over lateral part of tube

In Figure 19 a PGA No. 00 stitch fixes the wall of the tube to the uterine wall as shown at (1). The stitch holding the tube in the tunnel is seen at (2). In Figure 20 stitch (1) has been tied and a similar stitch is being used to close the open broad ligament between the divided ends of the tube (3). In Figure 21 the stitch covers the end of the lateral part of the tube so that there is no raw area or pedicle.

21

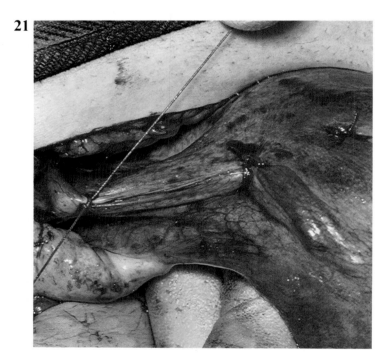

22

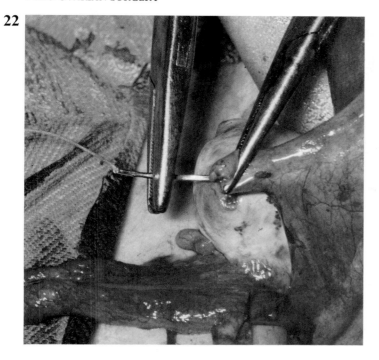

23

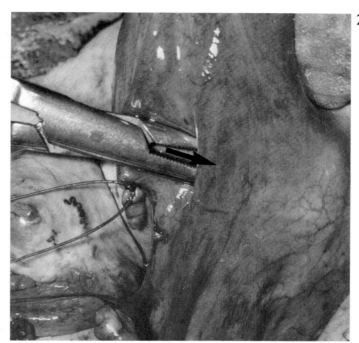

Procedure repeated on other side

22 to 25 Ligation and burying of right tube

A series of steps are repeated on the right side. The medial end of the tube is transfixed in Figure 22, the tunnel is prepared in Figure 23 along the line of the arrow and the tube (1) is introduced into the tunnel with the stitch ready to be tied (2) in

Figure 24. Figure 25 shows the tube being stitched to the uterus at its point of entry (1). The two layers of the broad ligament remain to be closed and in doing so, the cut and tied end of the lateral part of the tube (3) will be covered. This is effected by the suture which picks up the peritoneum at the two points (4) and (5).

24

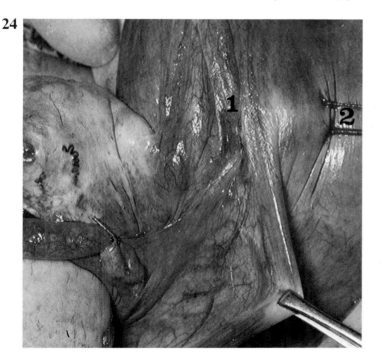

25

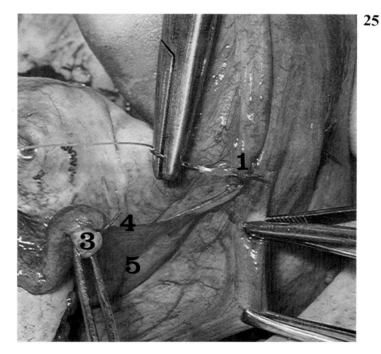

6: Endometriosis: conservative pelvic surgery including ventrosuspension

Despite the advent of improved progestational agents for the treatment of endometriosis, there remains a group of young women who require laparotomy. Many of these women are infertile and operation is planned to remove an endometriotic cyst which is causing tubal blockage, or to correct uterine retroversion. In some, continuing pain is an additional factor while in others it is the primary complaint at least at the time. Temporary relief of symptoms can be expected in most cases, although the success in relation to infertility is more questionable and almost impossible to compute. It must be expected that this type of surgery will sometimes be followed by recurrence of symptoms and many patients who had such conservative treatment are more than ready to accept hysterectomy in their early forties. If in the meantime they have achieved a pregnancy or pregnancies, the operation must be judged to have been a success.

The operation is carried out through a lower abdominal transverse incision. Adherent ovaries are freed and chocolate cysts excised or a partial oophorectomy is done on one or both ovaries. Endometriotic foci in the pouch of Douglas or over the attachments of the uterosacral ligaments are excised or fulgurated with a diathermy button; future retroversion of the uterus is prevented by doing a ventrosuspension operation.

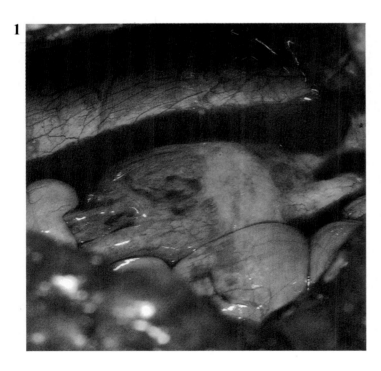

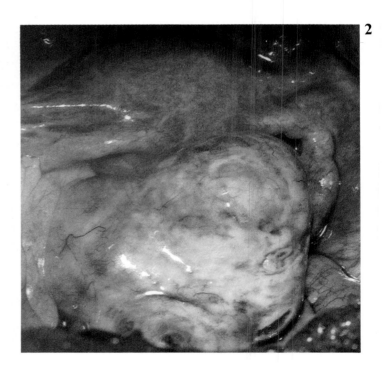

1 and 2 General view on opening abdomen

The typical picture of endometriosis is seen in Figure 1. There is some free fluid and the brown discolouration over the coils of bowel indicates the presence of old blood in the peritoneal cavity. The uterus itself is retroposed. In Figure 2 the fingers have hooked up the right ovary from the pouch of Douglas and it is seen to contain a chocolate cyst. The left ovary is not seen but contained a smaller chocolate cyst and was mobile.

Stage 1: Enucleation of endometriotic cyst

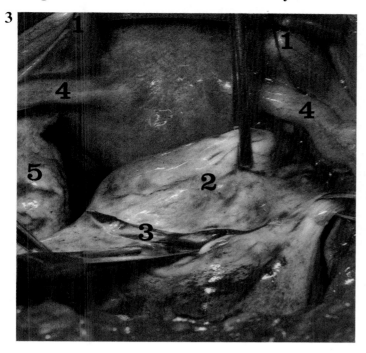

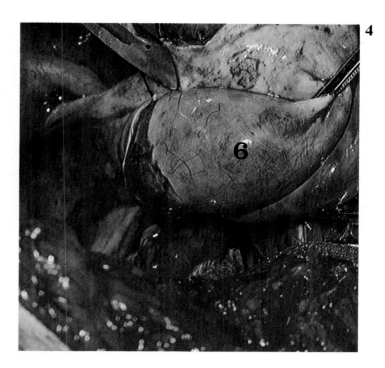

3 to 6 Enucleation of endometriotic cyst from right ovary

The uterus is held forward by stay sutures on the round ligaments (1) and (1) in Figure 3 and the ovarian capsule (2) is incised round the dome of the cyst to expose its wall (3). The tubes (4) and (4) and the enlarged left ovary (5) are seen. In Figure 4 the outline incision on the ovary includes a corpus luteum cyst (6) and Figure 5 gives a closer view posteriorly. In Figure 6 the cyst with the accompanying corpus luteum is ready to be detached from the ovary where arrowed.

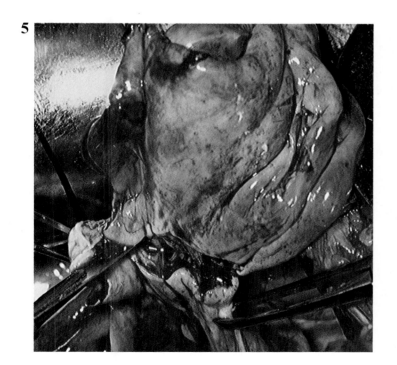

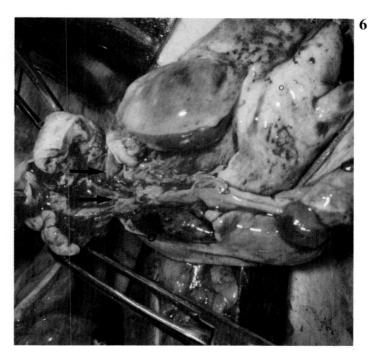

Stage 2: Reconstitution of ovary

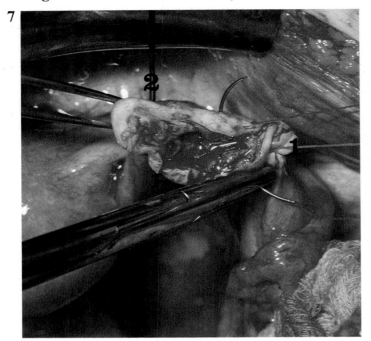

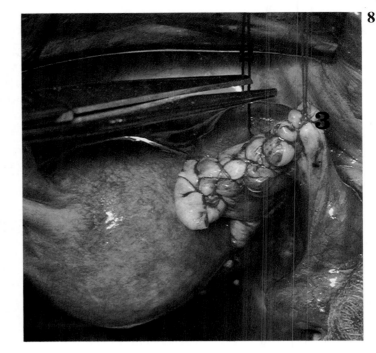

7 Reconstituting right ovary (1)

A certain amount of ovarian tissue has necessarily been removed with the chocolate cyst but about one-half of the ovary remains and the open surface presents as a V-shaped narrow trench. This is closed in the long axis of the ovary by inserting an over-and-over PGA No. 00 suture with stitches at a distance of 0.5 cm from each other to bring together the edges and control bleeding. The end of the anchor stitch is left long and held at (1) while the ovary is held by tissue forceps and closed transversely as shown. The stay suture on the right round ligament is numbered (2).

8 Reconstituting right ovary (2)

The same suture returns along the closed incision taking a more superficial bite of tissue at each stitch to ensure neat approximation of the edges and by an X effect with the stitches of the first suture line secures complete haemostasis. The ends of the stitch have been tied together at (3) and are about to be cut short. The stay suture on the right round ligament is still visible (2).

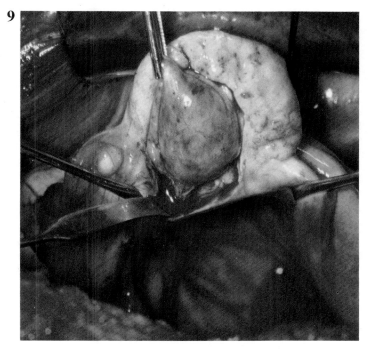

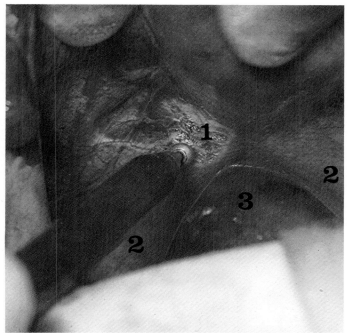

9 Enucleation of cyst from left ovary

The endometriotic cyst in the left ovary is being shelled out in routine fashion and the ovary will be reconstituted as described above.

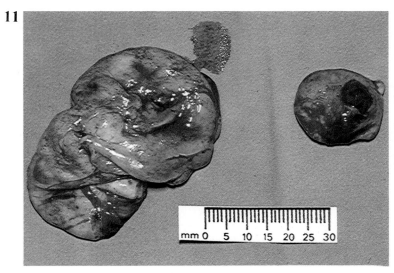

Stage 3: Treatment of endometriosis on peritoneum

10 Diathermy coagulation of area of endometriosis

Areas of endometriosis at the attachment of the uterosacral ligament or in the pouch of Douglas pose the question of how best to treat them. If there is much distortion of tissue and evidence of blood collection, the area should be excised and this was seen in the case of endometriosis treated by hysterectomy (page 95). If hysterectomy is not being carried out, the peritoneal plaque of endometriosis can be outlined superficially with the scalpel and dissected off the underlying structures. The surrounding peritoneum is freed peripherally if necessary and drawn together with fine stitches to cover the raw area.

In lesser degrees, as here, and where there are multiple small endometriotic spots or foci, the usual treatment is to fulgurate the areas with diathermy. A button electrode is very suitable and is seen in use (1) in the photograph. The uterosacral ligaments are numbered (2) and the pouch of Douglas (3).

11 Specimen

The collapsed larger chocolate cyst from the right ovary is seen on the left; it is almost impossible to remove these cysts without rupture. The small cyst from the left ovary is also shown.

Ventrosuspension

Until quite recently ventrosuspension was a common gynaecological operation. The majority of the women had mobile retroversion and backache. Unfortunately these symptoms tended to persist after operation; it is now considered essential to show that correction of the retroversion by a pessary relieves the backache before operating in this group.

The operation, however, has always been looked on as having a necessary part in conservative surgery of endometriosis. The uterus is usually retroposed and sometimes fixed in retroversion by fibrosis at the uterosacral attachments and by rectal adhesions. Patients with endometriosis suffer from dyspareunia in addition to backache; this is always more troublesome if retroversion is marked. The reasons for doing ventrosuspension in this group are apparently sound.

Simple plication of the round ligaments can lead to bowel adhesion at the site with subsequent obstruction and is not advised. The operation described is safe, permanent and can be recommended. The general aim is to obtain anteversion without undue tension on the round ligaments and with minimal trauma to the abdominal wall. There should be no residual raw areas or traps for the bowel which could cause future complications. The details are described in the text.

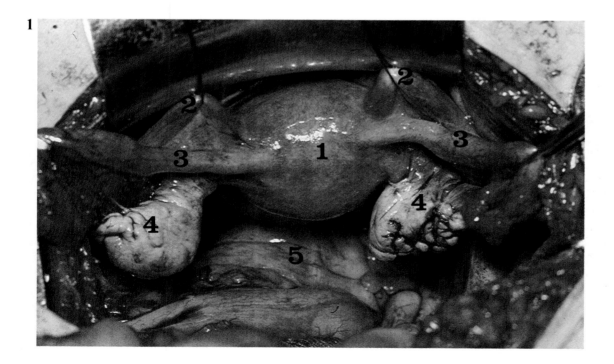

1 General appearance before ventrosuspension

The illustration shows the structures at the end of the operation just described: (1) uterus, (2) round ligaments, (3) fallopian tubes, (4) ovaries, (5) rectum. The uterus is not retroverted but is retroposed and is being held forwards by the stay sutures on the round ligaments. These sutures were purposely placed 1.5 cm from the body of the uterus and encircling the whole ligament so that they could subsequently be used as tractors to bring the round ligaments extraperitoneally to be fixed to the anterior rectus sheath.

Stage 1: Preparation of route for round ligaments

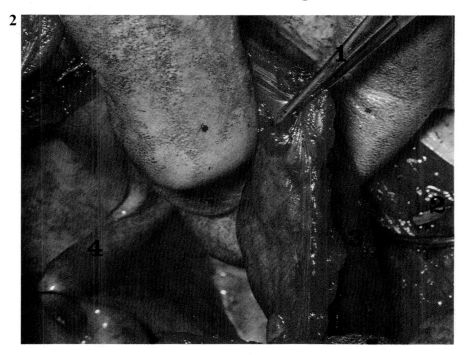

2 Preparing route for right round ligament (1)

With fine forceps (1) on the peritoneal edge and tissue forceps (2) on the edge of the rectus sheath the surgeon picks up the whole right rectus muscle belly (3) between his forefinger and thumb. The right round ligament with its suture is numbered (4).

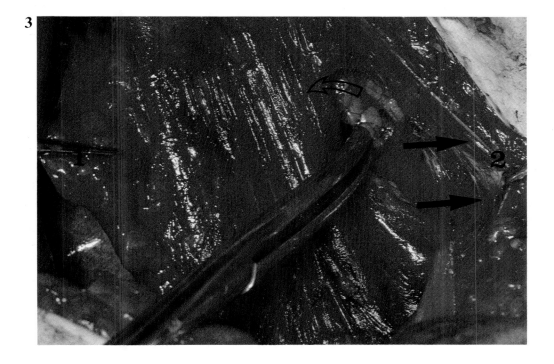

3 Preparing route for right round ligament (2)

Keeping the peritoneal edge (1) taut medially and the rectus sheath (2) laterally as arrowed, a round ligament (or Phillips) forceps is introduced lateral to the muscle ready to travel extraperitoneally towards the suture on the right round ligament in the direction of the arrow. Care is taken to avoid the inferior epigastric blood vessels which would cause a haematoma if damaged.

4

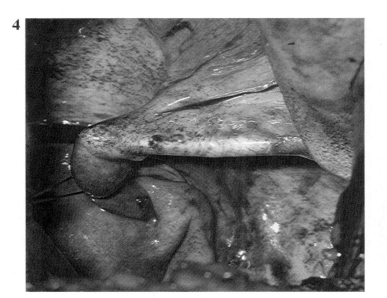

5

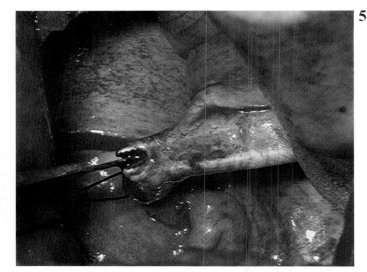

4 to 7 Preparing extraperitoneal path for right round ligament

The forceps are passed extraperitoneally towards the inguinal ring initially and then medially and upwards along the line of the round ligament and as shown in Figure 4. The points of the forceps are under direct vision during their journey and kept superficial and clear of blood vessels. In Figure 5 the jaws are opened and the stretched peritoneum incised. In Figure 6 the end of the suture on the round ligament is fed on to the forceps which will be withdrawn in the direction of the arrow. In Figure 7 the forceps have been withdrawn and still holding the suture to bring the apex of the round ligament loop into the rectus sheath lateral to the muscle at (1).

6

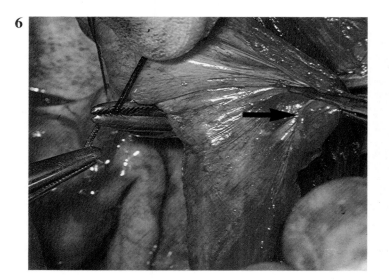

7

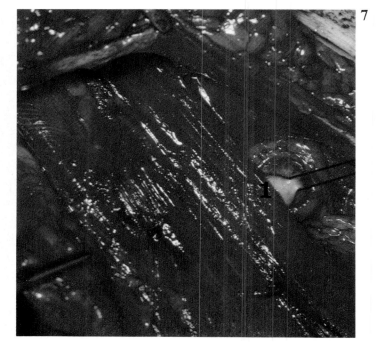

Stage 2: Retrieval of round ligaments

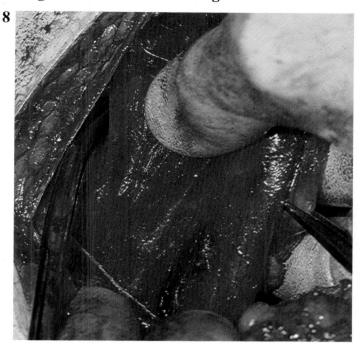

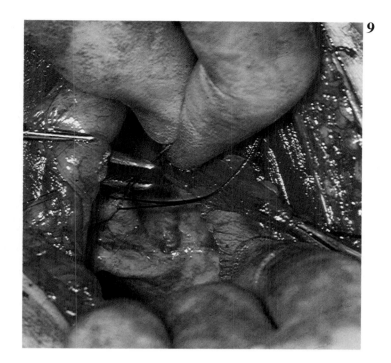

8 to 11 Retrieval of left round ligament

The same steps are repeated on the left side, in Figures 8, 9 and 10, leaving the knuckle of the left round ligament at point (1). In Figure 11 the lower leaf of the rectus sheath is retracted with tissue forceps (1) and the peritoneal edge is drawn back with small artery forceps (2) to show the fundus of the uterus (3) and the left round ligament (4) drawn laterally and extraperitoneally by its attached suture in the direction of the arrow.

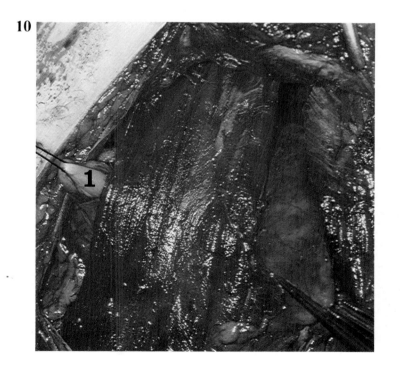

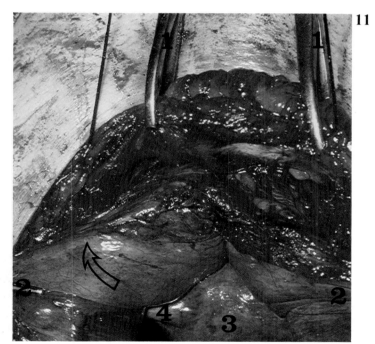

12

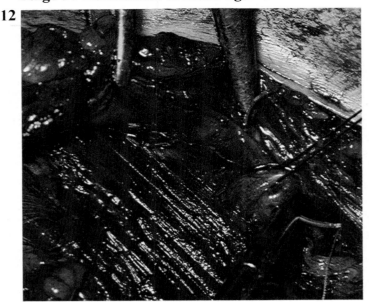

13

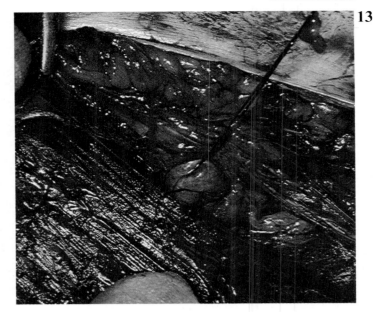

12 to 15 Attaching right round ligament to rectus sheath

In Figure 12 the needle carrying a PGA No. 0 suture pierces both limbs of the round ligament loop and then picks up the lower leaf of the anterior rectus sheath at least 2 cm clear of its cut edge. In Figure 13 the stitch is tied and in Figure 14 it is cut short and a second suture is being placed close to it. In Figure 15 the tractor suture has been removed from the round ligament and the second attaching stitch is tied and ready to be cut short.

14

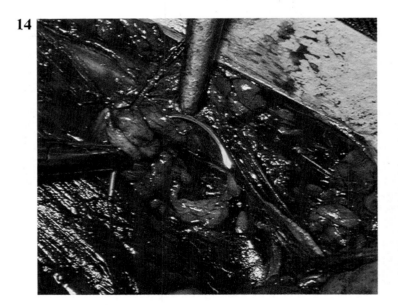

15

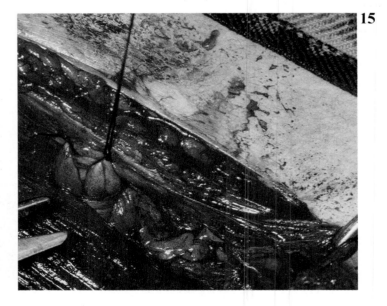

16

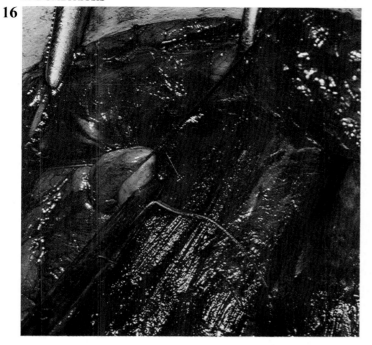

17

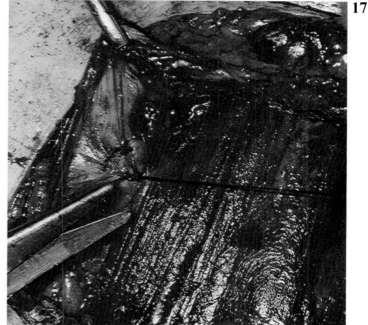

16 and 17 Attaching left round ligament to rectus sheath

Two stages in the same procedure are shown on the left side. The knuckle of the round ligament is firmly but not tightly sutured to the sheath to avoid traumatising it. The authors would like to mention without comment three certain cases they know of where a localised endometrioma developed at the site of round ligament fixation and had to be excised. Catgut suture was used in all instances and nothing untoward was reported at the time of the operation.

18

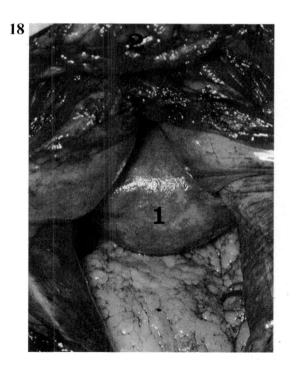

19

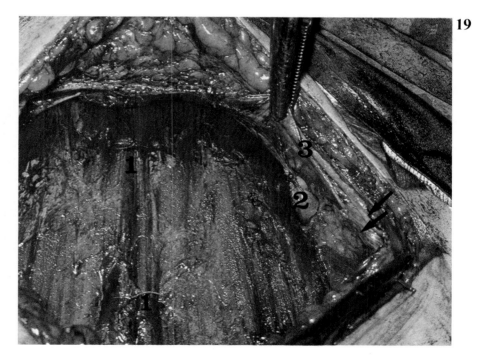

18 Uterus drawn into anteversion

The peritoneal edges are pulled laterally to show how the uterus (1) has been drawn forwards towards the symphysis pubis (2) by the repositioned round ligaments.

19 Rectus sheath ready for closure

The recti muscles have been approximated in the midline by two stitches (1) and (1) and the knuckle of the right round ligaments (2) is seen attached to the lower leaf of the rectus sheath quite clear of the cut edge (3). The two layers of the rectus sheath (arrowed) are being picked up by a stitch which indicates the start of its closure. The appearance on the left side is similar.

7: Operation for acute pelvic inflammatory disease

Though the incidence of acute pelvic inflammation is enormously reduced, cases are still seen following septic abortion or gonococcal and non-specific genital infection. Nearly all such cases are treated with antibiotics in the first place and the gynaecologist hopes and finds that in most situations operation can be avoided. However, severe degrees are still commonplace in developing countries and there is less prospect of treating these conservatively. It is not proposed to refer to cases in older women where a ruptured diverticular or malignant abscess causes peritonitis. Their presentation and management is quite different.

Despite what has been said laparotomy sometimes becomes mandatory and if not done can lead to the patient's death. Response to powerful and different antibiotics may be unsatisfactory or the condition obviously progresses to peritonitis. In most cases, however, a combination of factors forces the surgeon's hand. In such clinical situations the patient is desperately ill with a high swinging temperature and a fast pulse and is not apparently responding to any antibiotic. There is abdominal distention with absence of bowel sounds and a mass in the pelvis. One cannot be certain that the condition had not arisen from a ruptured appendix. As the patient's condition worsens, there is the risk of missing the chance of doing laparotomy. This was exactly the position in the case to be described. Inevitably in such circumstances laparotomy has to be done.

The procedure is set out in the text, but the authors wish to emphasise that in this condition surgical intervention is only a part of the treatment and is being used for two specific purposes. The first is to exclude or deal with any non-gynaecological condition such as appendiceal or diverticular abscess. The second is to treat any tubal lesion by ensuring adequate drainage and relief of tension and so allow nature to complete the recovery. There has been a tendency to meddle with and remove inflamed tubes and even ovaries. This is unnecessary and leads to irremedial sterility. In a proportion of very severe cases treated by drainage and antibiotics fertility has survived; in others there has at least been a basis on which future treatment could build hopefully. Once the pus has been found and drained adequately, and if the patient has been spared operative shock and undue anaesthesia, recovery is usually rapid. Gastric suction, intravenous fluids, electrolyte balance and perhaps blood transfusion will no doubt all be required, but patients in this group are young and nearly always do well.

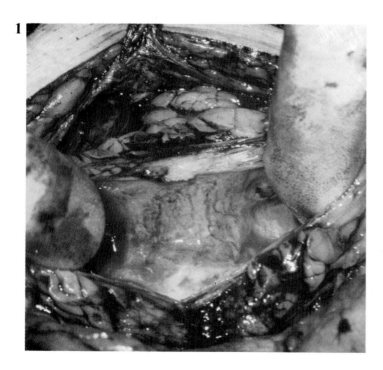
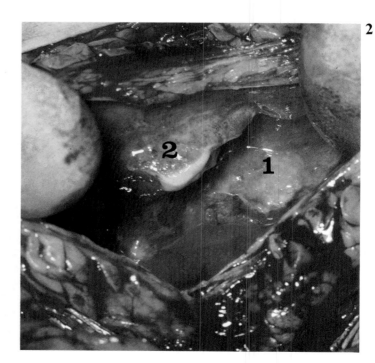

1 and 2 General view on opening abdomen

Oedema of all the structures and inflammatory exudate over and between the coils of bowel attached to the fundus of the uterus are seen in Figure 1. There is every evidence of locked off pus in the pelvis. In Figure 2 the fingers pull the wound edges apart more widely and the easily separated coils of bowel fall away to show the swollen appendages on the right (1) and on the left (2). The uterus itself is pushed forwards and is not visible.

Stage 1: Release of pus and mobilisation of appendages

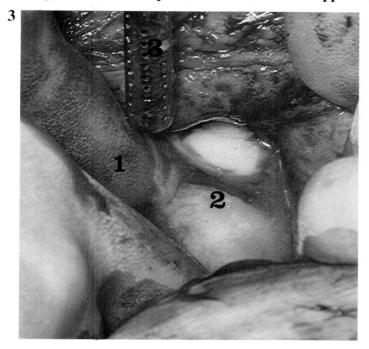

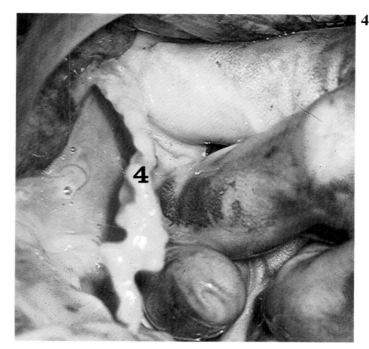

3 to 5 Release of pus from pelvis

In Figure 3 and after placing a large moist swab at the pelvic brim to prevent contamination of the abdomen, the surgeon's finger (1) gently probes behind the swollen appendages (2) towards the pouch of Douglas and a sucker (3) is kept ready for action. In Figure 4 pus gushes out (4) after separation of fine adhesions around the left appendages and quickly fills the wound. In Figure 5 the pus is shown being removed with the sucker and a throat swab (5) is seen obtaining a laboratory specimen of the pus for immediate culture and tests for sensitivity to antibiotic drugs.

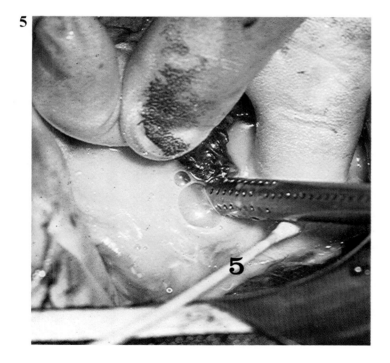

6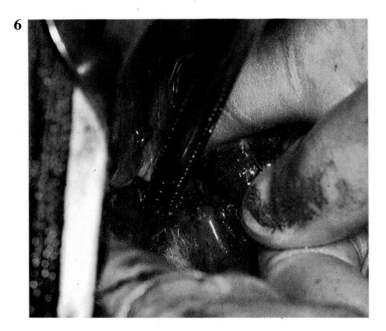

7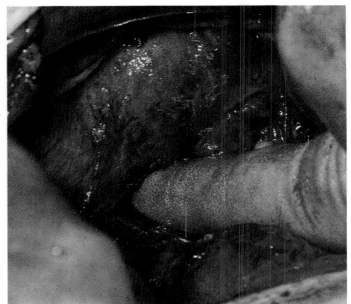

6 and 7 Release of appendages from pouch of Douglas

In Figure 6 the pus has largely been removed from the pelvis.
In Figure 7 the surgeon's finger gently releases and elevates the
swollen and inflamed appendages into the wound on the left
side.

8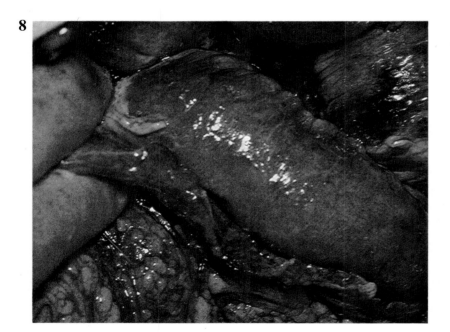

8 Release of coil of small intestine from pouch of Douglas

It was found that a loop of small intestine was adherent to the
pouch of Douglas; this is shown being milked free between
forefinger and thumb and will be restored to the abdomen.
The inflamed bowel is friable and easily torn. If this happens it
is immediately closed in two layers as described on page 111.

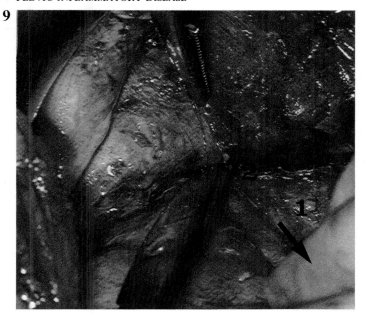

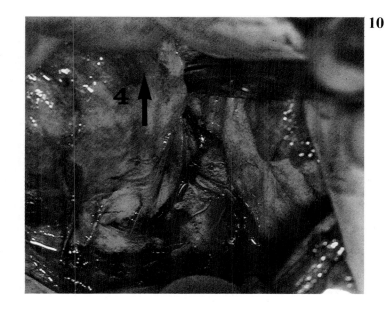

9 to 11 Exploration of pouch of Douglas

Because drainage must be from the depth of the pouch of Douglas, it is essential to explore the area and ensure that there are no remaining pockets of pus. In Figure 9 the right appendages (1) are being freed gently in the direction of the arrow where an adhesion has been divided (2). In Figure 10 the left appendages (4) are eased up in the direction of the arrow from the pelvic floor. In Figure 11 the surgeon's hand steadies uterus and appendages (5) forwards while reaching down to the pouch of Douglas. The sucker (6) is keeping the pelvis clear of pus.

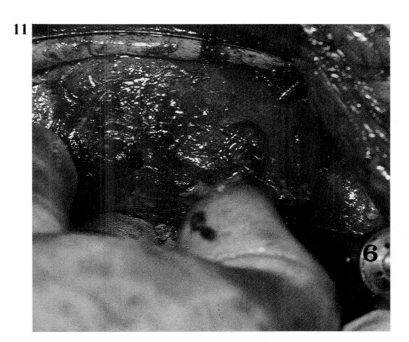

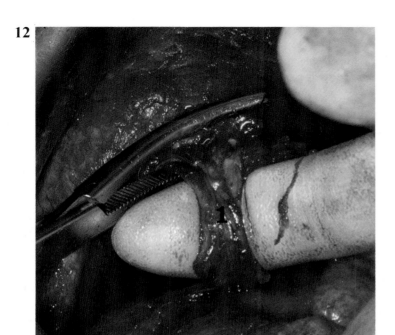

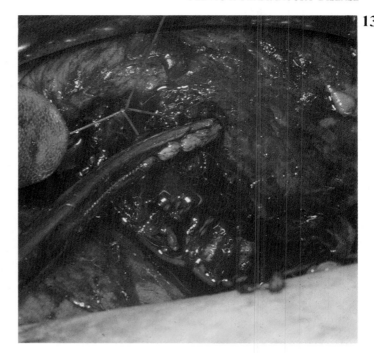

12 to 15 Further exploration of pouch of Douglas

It is not possible to lay down specific rules of technique in these cases because each is different, but the steps shown here are frequently required. A broad adhesion deep in the pelvis (1) between sigmoid colon and uterus is displayed and clamped in Figure 12. It is tied off in Figure 13 and frees the uterus and appendages considerably. The right tube (2) is separated from its adhesions in Figure 14 and is seen as a tense pyosalpinx. Figure 15 shows the uterus (3) anteriorly with the swollen right tube (2) and an empty cavity (4) in the region of the left tube. The latter was almost certainly the source of much of the pus as the abscess was around the tube on the left rather than within it.

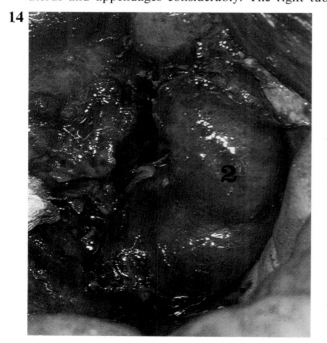

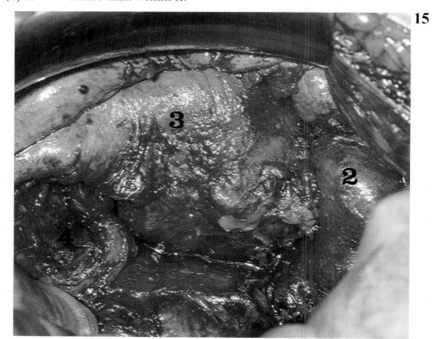

Stage 2: Drainage of pelvis

There are no particular advantages attached to any one type of drain. The aim is to keep a free and open track to the exterior; except in the case of a viscus the drainage is around rather than through the drain. Tubes tend to become blocked and for most purposes corrugated plastic is used. The type used is an attempt at a compromise.

The technique shown can be similarly used when the surgeon encounters other instances of lower abdominal collections of pus, such as in diverticular or appendiceal abscesses.

16 to 20 Drainage of pelvis

This sequence of figures shows the various steps in the insertion of Ragnell drains, one on each side of the pelvis and being brought out through the lateral aspect of the transverse wound. The type of drain is shown in Figure 16; an opening into the peritoneal cavity is made lateral to the left rectus muscle in Figure 17 and opened up in Figure 18 at (1). A sinus forceps draws the outer end of the left pelvic drain through the opening in Figures 19 and 20, in the direction of the arrow.

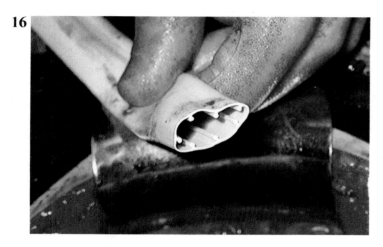

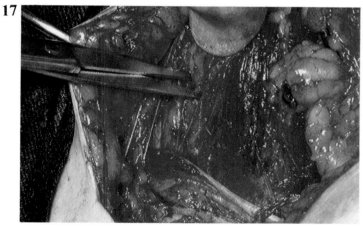

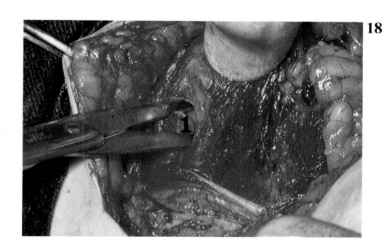

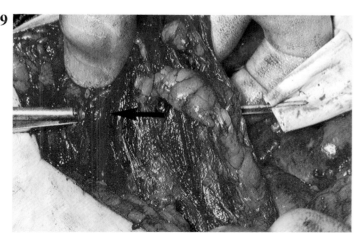

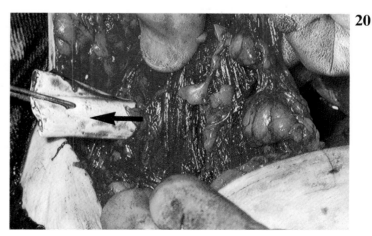

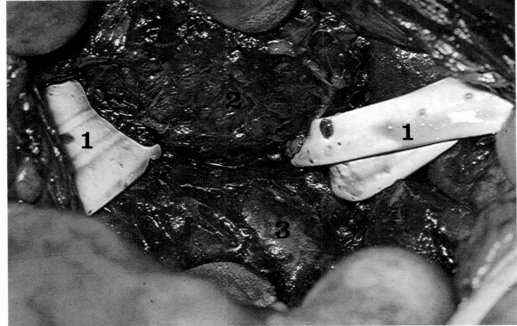

21 Pelvic drains shown in place

The two drains (1) and (1) which extend to the depth of the pelvis behind the uterus and appendages (2) are seen in place and fanning out towards their exit points on each side. The rectum is seen posteriorly (3).

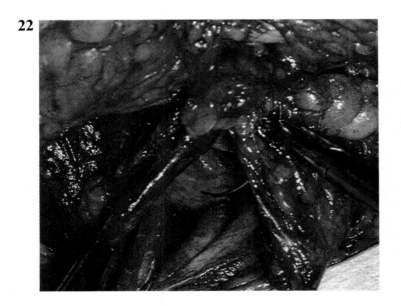

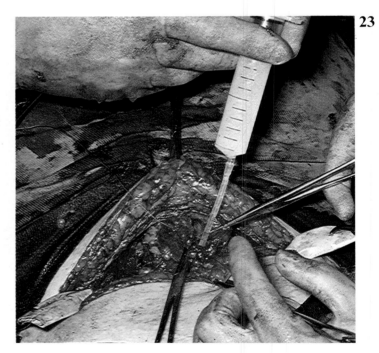

22 and 23 Closure of peritoneal cavity and installation of antibiotic intraperitoneally

Closure of the peritoneal layers with a PGA No. 0 suture commences at the upper end of the wound in Figure 22 and in Figure 23 100 ml of *Noxythiolin (2.5 per cent sol) is injected into the peritoneal cavity before the closing stitch is tied off.

*A white crystalline powder, 2.5 g noxythiolin, 10 mg amethocaine Hcl BP.

24

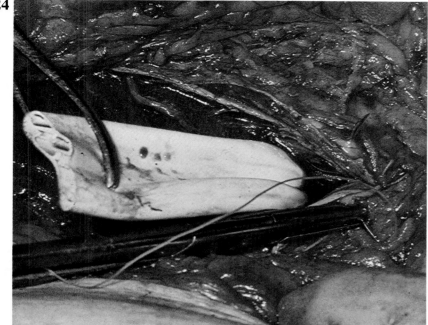

24 Positioning of pelvic drains in wound
It is undesirable to have the drain in the angle of
the rectus sheath where the two layers are open
to possible spread of infection. Two sutures are
first placed lateral to each drain as shown and
the rectus sheath is then closed transversely
between the drains.

25

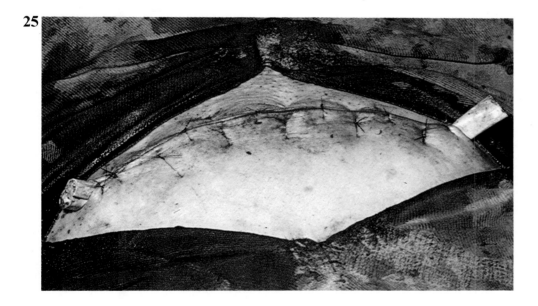

25 Skin closure
The wound is seen closed by a series of vertical mattress
sutures and intermediate small sutures to make skin edge
approximation neat. The drains are seen in the angles of the
wound. The stitches are of monofilmament nylon and are tied
just sufficiently tight to give good approximation of the skin
edges.

8: Appendicectomy

The inclusion of appendicectomy in this volume of the Atlas and the reasons for doing so have been referred to in the Introduction. Apart from strictly medical indications there is always the question of whether a gynaecologist should look on appendicectomy as a procedure which ought to be added to a straightforward pelvic operation. Hysterectomy, ovariotomy and ventrosuspension represent the type of case in question.

Clearly the decision depends entirely on the circumstances and it would require a volume to pursue the hypothetical possibilities. The authors offer one defensive piece of advice to the surgeon under criticism for not having done the operation. To remove the appendix entails opening the bowel with the possibility of infection of the operative field and all the dangers that may arise from such an occurrence.

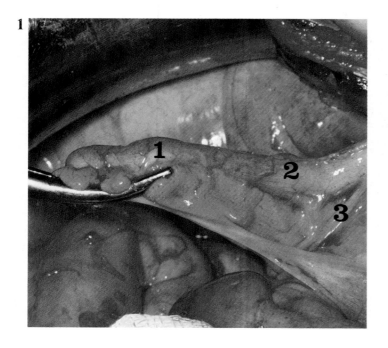

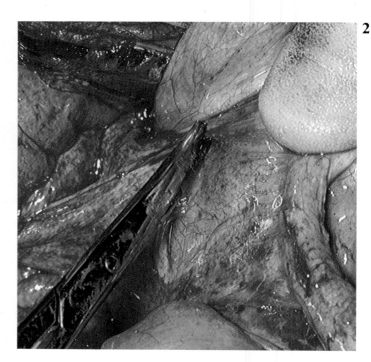

1 Appearance of inflamed appendix

The appendix is long, thickened and obviously inflamed. The wall is oedematous with small blood vessel coursing over its surface. Faecoliths are easily palpable at (1) and (2) and the appendix is partially kinked by a peritoneal band at (3).

2 Division of peritoneal adhesions

It is nearly always necessary to divide peritoneal adhesions or folds to mobilise the appendix and gain access to its mesentery. That is being done with the scissors in this illustration.

Stage 1: Division of mesentery

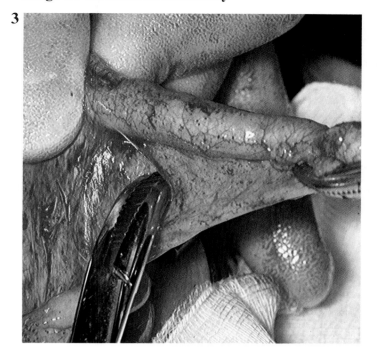

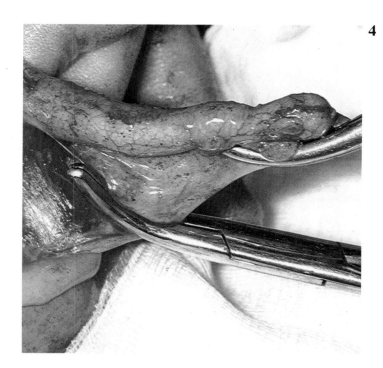

3 to 5 Clamping and dividing mesentery of appendix (1)

In Figure 3 the appendix is lifted between the finger and thumb at its midpoint to show the mesentery and its tip is held by a Phillips forceps on the mesenteric edge. A similar forceps is used to make an opening in the mesentery before clamping the first part. In Figure 4 a first clamping forceps is applied to grasp the mesentery as far as the opening made in it; in Figure 5 the distal part of the appendix is being detached with scissors. Note that a good cuff of tissue is left beyond the jaws of the forceps.

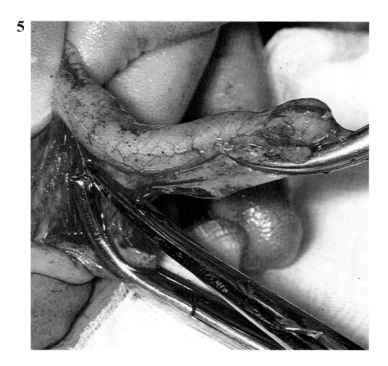

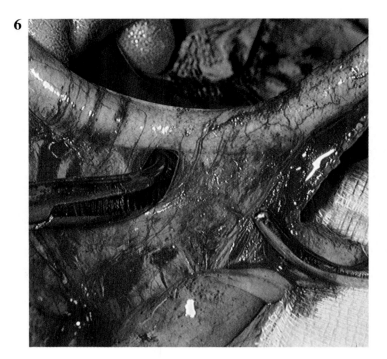

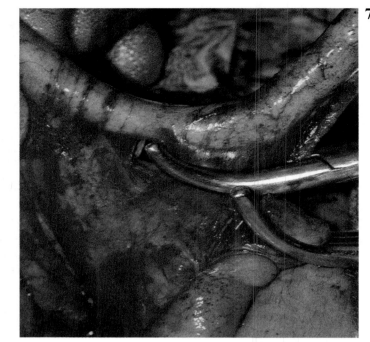

6 and 7 Clamping and dividing mesentery of appendix (2)
The same procedure is carried out with a second bite of mesentery and leaves the appendix almost fully separated.

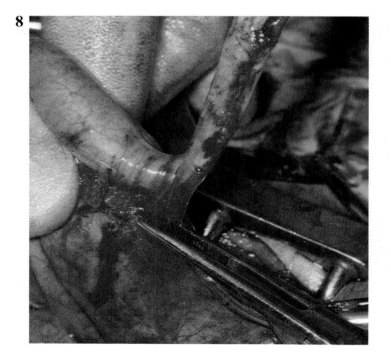

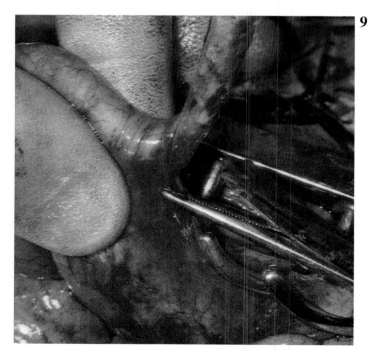

8 and 9 Securing artery to the appendix
The main branch of the artery to the appendix runs parallel to it within the mesoappendix and sends branches around it. The vessel enters the mesentery in the angle which has now been reached and it is important that it be definitively secured with fine artery forceps as shown in Figure 8. If it is not dealt with at this stage, removal of the appendix is awkward because it is not fully released; as a result the artery may be torn or damaged and cause bleeding or haematoma. Figure 9 shows the vessel clamped safely and the appendix completely free of its mesentery.

Stage 2: Removal of appendix

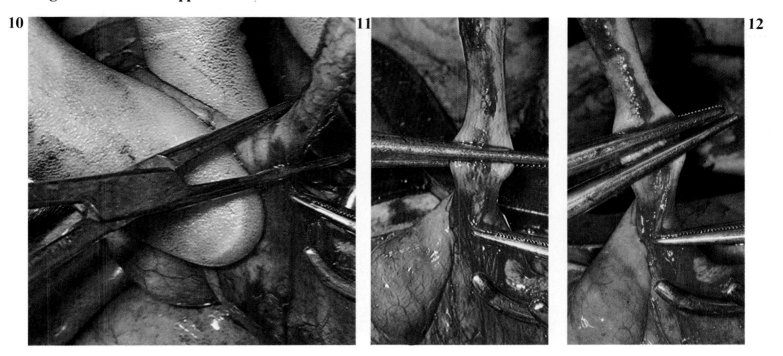

10 to 15 Crushing, clamping and removing appendix

In Figure 10 the appendix is crushed with heavy forceps close to the caecum in an area where it will be ligated subsequently. In Figure 11 the forceps are reapplied more distally on what will be the stump of the appendix. A second forceps is applied distal and close to it in Figure 12 and the appendix detached between them by sliding the scalpel along the surface of the first forceps, as in Figure 13. In Figure 14 the appendix with its holding forceps and the soiled scalpel are all consigned to a

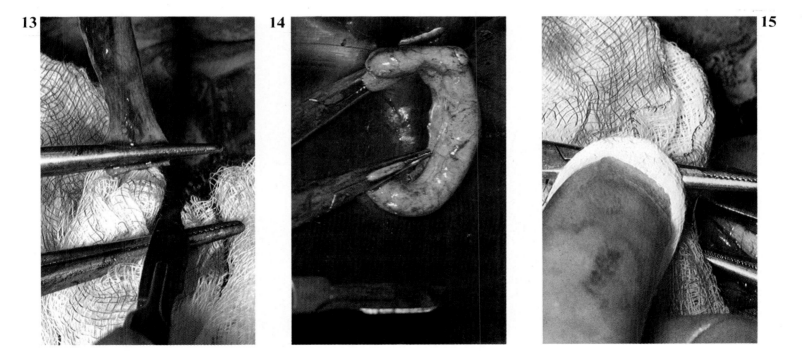

container for soiled instruments. In Figure 15 the cut end of the stump is wiped clean with a swab along the jaws of the holding forceps. The swab joins the soiled instruments and is removed from the operation field.

16
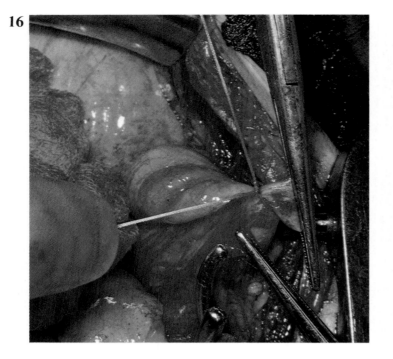

17
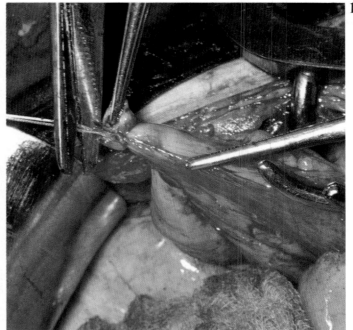

16 to 19 Ligation of appendix stump and mesenteric pedicles

In Figure 16 the appendix stump is ligated with PGA No. 0 suture in the previously crushed area. The tip of this stump is then held with fine forceps and the suture cut as in Figure 17. In Figure 18 PGA No. 00 suture is used to tie the appendicular artery: in Figure 19 the inner mesenteric pedicle (1) is tied with the same suture material. The outer mesenteric pedicle (2) is then similarly dealt with.

18
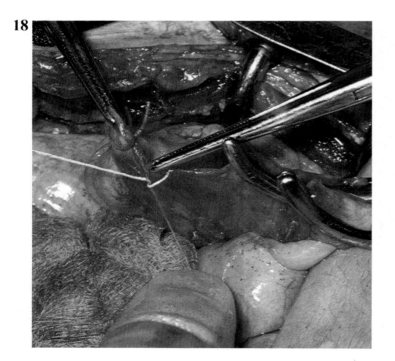

19
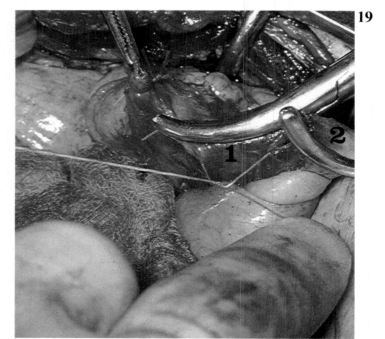

Stage 3: Purse string suture

20

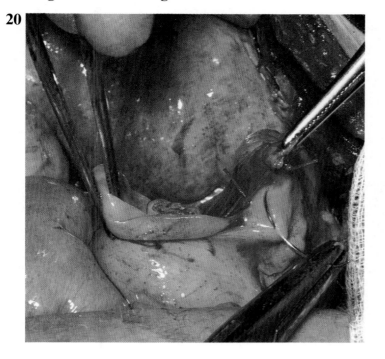

21

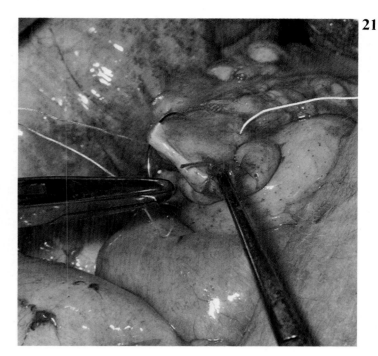

20 to 22 Insertion of purse string suture

With the ligated appendix stump held in the fine forceps, stages in the placement of a purse string of PGA No. 00 suture are shown in Figures 20, 21 and 22. Vessels are obviously avoided with the needle and especially in the region of the mesoappendix.

22

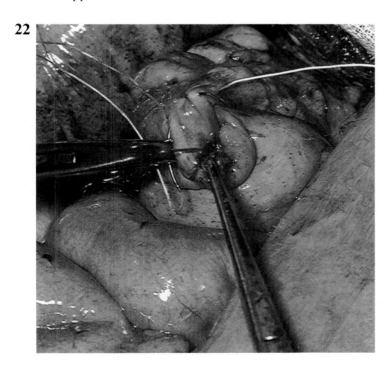

23
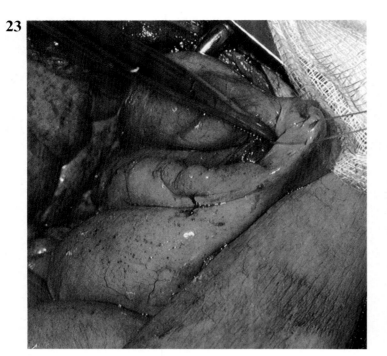

24
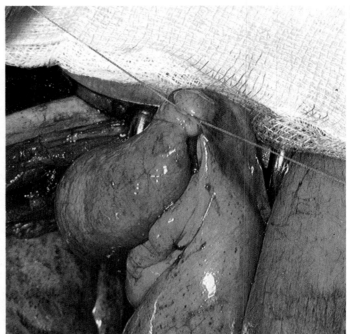

23 and 24 Covering stump of appendix

In Figure 23 the ends of the purse-string suture are drawn up tight, while the assistant inverts the tip of the appendix so that it is buried underneath the peritoneum as the suture is drawn tight. The stitch is seen being tied off in Figure 24.

9: Laparoscopy

Laparoscopy has developed as a valuable and almost indispensable surgical technique during the last decade. Gynaecologists had realised the benefits of pelvic endoscopy with culdoscopy but the knee-chest position gave anaesthetic and other problems and fibreoptic systems were not then available. The modern laparoscope is a valuable diagnostic and operating tool which now has an established place in gynaecological surgery. General abdominal surgeons are beginning to realise its potential advantages to them and there seems little doubt that the laparoscope will be used increasingly for upper abdominal as well as pelvic work.

Applications in gynaecology

Originally conceived and used as a purely diagnostic procedure, laparoscopy has been developed increasingly in gynaecology for diathermy and other forms of sterilisation. It is now estimated that in fact more than half of all laparoscopies done in the United Kingdom are for female sterilisation. In the following text the techniques for these two applications of laparoscopy will be considered separately and in detail. It is not proposed to deal with the more specialised uses such as in ovarian biopsy, ventrosuspension of the uterus and assessment of pelvic malignancy.

Laparoscopy as a diagnostic method has two main applications. The first is in relation to the investigation of infertility and the second is in the differential diagnosis of abdominal and pelvic pain. With regard to the former it is possible to make a complete visual examination of uterus, tubes and ovaries and at the same time test tubal patency by injecting dye through the cervix and along the tubes to the peritoneal cavity. The cause of pelvic pain whether acute or chronic is often a matter of doubt and anxiety to the gynaecologist and laparoscopy has eased many of the problems. The acute case of a possible ectopic pregnancy or tubal infection or even appendicitis can be solved in a few minutes without opening the abdomen, while the patient with chronic pelvic pain can either be accorded the diagnostic dignity of having pelvic endometriosis or be shown to have no overt or obviously dangerous pelvic pathology.

Sterilisation through the laparoscope may be done in several ways and these will be considered in detail in the text under the appropriate heading. There must obviously be problems in relation to the use of diathermy current within the peritoneal cavity and the risks of burning the viscera. Therefore, it is not surprising that alternative non-diathermy methods have been sought and developed, but diathermy coagulation is still the principal method used and the problems related to it have to be faced.

When a new method like laparoscopy is so universally useful it is essential to look to its safety and instructions on how to avoid complications will be given in the text as required.

When laparoscopy is used for diagnosis dangers are relatively few, but the use of the diathermy electrode in sterilisation has led to bowel and other damage which is very worrying. The National Survey of 1977 organised by the Royal College of Obstetricians and Gynaecologists sets out the situation as found in the United Kingdom today. One can do no better than refer readers to their reports which are generally reassuring. As far as the clinical procedure is concerned, most gynaecologists find themselves clumsy with the laparoscope initially but the technique is learned quickly and becomes very easy. The moral is that safe laparoscopy depends very much on the operator having been trained properly and experienced in the method. Once practised in the technique there is even an understandable tendency to use it in cutting clinical corners.

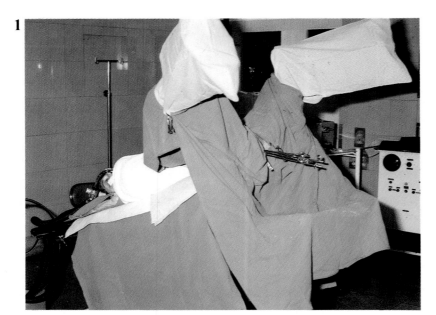

1 Patient prepared for laparoscopy

The patient is in the lithotomy and moderate Trendelenburg position. The bladder has been emptied and an intrauterine catheter is in position, as she is a case for investigation of infertility. The patient is of course intubated and maintained on artificial respiration.

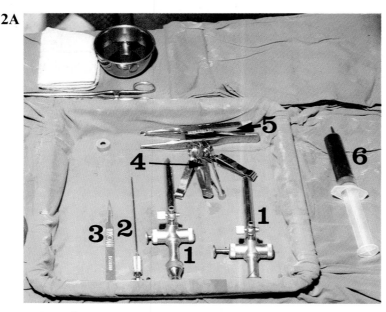

2A and 2B Laparoscopic equipment

The items in Figure 2A are essentially those used for introduction of the instrument into the peritoneal cavity and include:

1 Trochar and cannula
2 Verres needle
3 Sharp pointed scalpel
4 Towel clips
5 Michel clip forceps
6 Methylene blue dye to determine tubal patency

The items in Figure 2B are those used in laparoscopic examination biopsy and sterilisation and include:

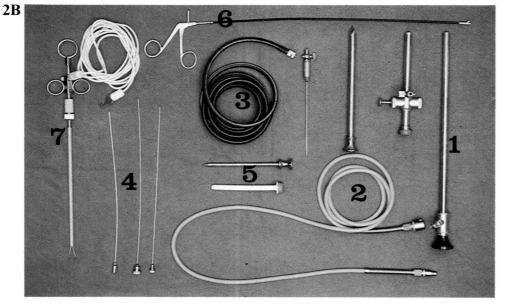

1 Examining telescope
2 Fibreoptic cable
3 CO_2 gas tube
4 Stilette needles as probes or for aspiration
5 Trochar and cannula for second portal
6 Ovarian biopsy forceps
7 Diathermy forceps

3

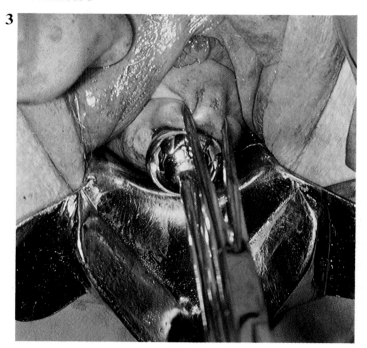

3 Intrauterine cannula fixed in position

The cone-shaped end of the Spackman cannula is held firmly in the cervical canal by a locked attachment to the volsellum placed on the anterior lip of the cervix.

4

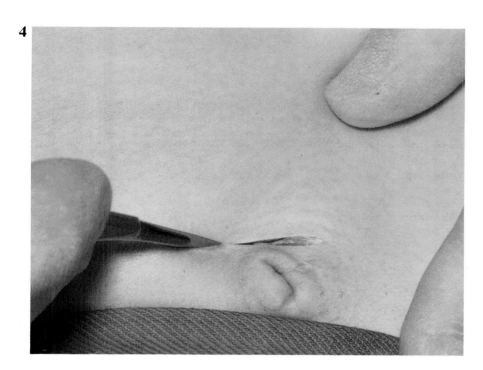

4 Skin incision

This incision is made just on the lower edge of the umbilicus to the depth of the rectus sheath and is about 2 cm long.

237

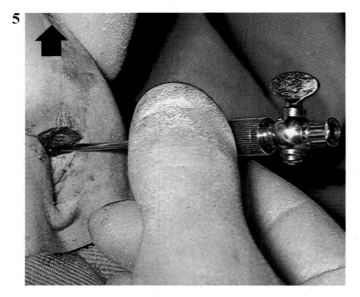

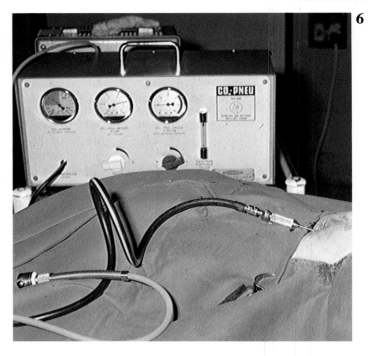

5 Insertion of Verres needle

The Verres needle has a spring-loaded and perforated blunt trochar within a sharp cannula to avoid visceral damage. Holding and lifting upwards (as arrowed) the loose tissues of the lower abdominal wall in the left hand, the needle is introduced clear of the sacral promentary towards the coccyx. It is felt to traverse first the rectus sheath and then the peritoneum during insertion.

6 Recording intra-abdominal pressure

With the gas flow coupled up to the Verres needle, the intra-abdominal pressure is carefully observed on the pressure dial of the laparoscope monitor. The pressure should not exceed 15 to 20 mmHg and if it does this indicates that the end of the needle is probably not free in the peritoneal cavity and the needle should be re-inserted. The probability would be that it was in a viscus or extraperitoneal and would not therefore show oscillations with respiration. The pressures too would tend to build up.

7 Observation of gas flow and volume

The right-hand dial of the laparoscope monitor shows the intra-abdominal pressure and the left-hand dial the volume of gas introduced into the peritoneal cavity. The carbon dioxide is run in at a speed of 1 litre/min; the amount used is very much a question of the surgeon's individual preference. The authors prefer about 3 litres of gas.

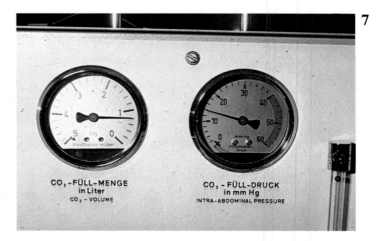

8

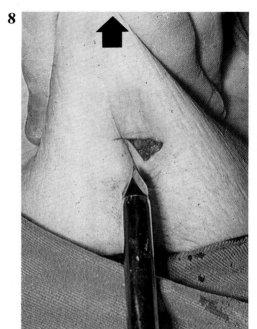

9

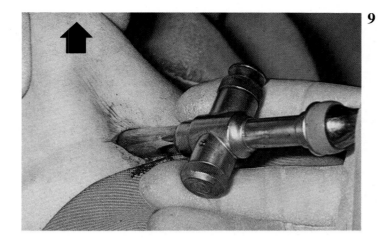

8 to 11 Insertion of laparoscope

The Trendelenburg position is increased steeply at this stage and with the loose tissues of the lower abdomen held in the left hand as shown in Figure 8 the surgeon prepares to insert the trochar and cannula. The anterior abdominal wall is elevated firmly. It is generally preferable to have made a small incision in the rectus sheath with the scalpel so as to make entry easier. In Figure 9 the trochar is shown being inserted by a pushing and partially rotating movement and perforation of the abdominal wall is easily recognised. The direction of insertion is again towards the coccyx and the trochar and cannula traverse the abdominal wall obliquely. In Figure 10 the trochar has been removed and the CO_2 insufflation tube has been connected. The cannula valve is depressed and a rush of gas indicates to the surgeon that the cannula is in the peritoneal cavity. The cannula allows the telescope to enter when the valve is depressed and in Figure 11 it is seen in place. The CO_2 control knob is being opened to keep up the intra-abdominal pressure by a slow flow of 250 ml/min of gas.

10

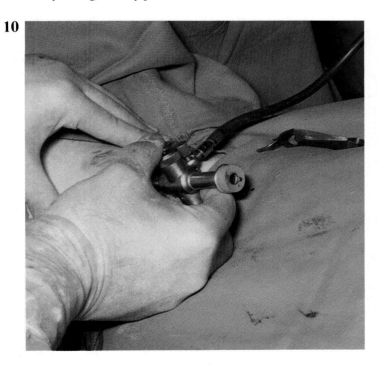

11

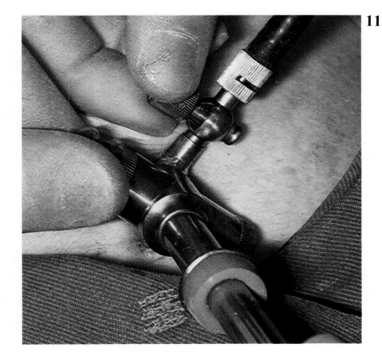

239

12

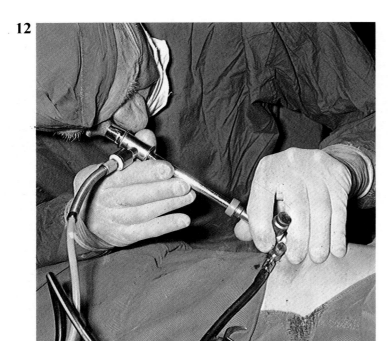

13

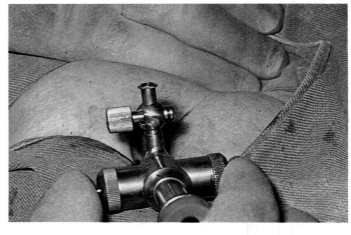

14

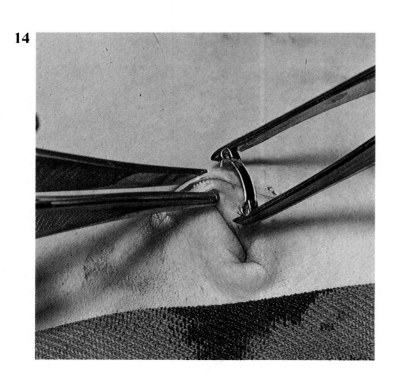

12 Laparoscopic examination

Examination is made in the manner shown in the illustration. The tip of the endoscope is passed through some warm water and a drop of glycerine applied to it before entry to avoid clouding when in the peritoneal cavity. If clouding occurs during examination, it can usually be dispersed by holding the end of the telescope against a coil of bowel for a few seconds. There are two examining telescopes: a direct viewing and a right-angled viewing one. During examination it is frequently necessary to manipulate the viscera to get an adequate view and a palpateur or probe is introduced through the abdominal wall at the lateral border of the right rectus muscle just below the level of the umbilicus after making a nick in the skin with the sharp pointed scalpel. Biopsy forceps or other larger instruments require a trochar and cannula puncture as in sterilisation laparoscopy. Transillumination of the abdominal wall with the endoscope during insertion of the small trochar and cannula enables one to avoid blood vessels, i.e. inferior epigastric.

13 Expulsion of gas from peritoneal cavity

After examination and removal of the telescope the valve on the cannula is depressed and gas is forced out of the pelvis and lower abdomen by manual pressure as shown. The cannula is then withdrawn.

14 Skin closure

Two narrow clips or a subcuticular stitch are equally suitable for closing the skin.

Laparoscopic sterilisation procedures

The usual procedure and essentially the one reviewed in the National Survey is tubal coagulation by unipolar diathermy. This is likely to be the method used for several years to come and is described below. Single portal operating laparoscopes are now available, but any advantages of having laparoscopic and diathermy forceps in the one instrument seem to be cancelled out by loss of flexibility in having telescope and instrument combined.

The complication rate from burns is about three per cent; it has been suggested that this might be reduced by using bipolar diathermy where the patient is excluded from the electric circuit. On the other hand it might not be so efficient because the area of the burn is necessarily very localised. When tubal diathermy was first used it was considered necessary to divide the tube after its coagulation, but this step was subsequently seen to be the chief cause of postoperative intraperitoneal bleeding from the vessels of the mesosalpinx while adding nothing to the effectiveness of the procedure. It has now been abandoned.

It is generally accepted that laparoscopic tubal diathermy should not be done in the puerperium because of the height of the fundus, general vascularity and dangers of bleeding. Postabortal sterilisation is done on a large scale for reasons of expediency, but the dangers should be kept in mind; special care must be taken to avoid the fundus of the uterus with the Verres needle and the trochar. The inevitably vascular tubes should be handled carefully with the forceps to avoid bleeding from vessels in the mesosalpinx and division of the tube should certainly be avoided.

In laparoscopic as in any other form of sterilisation preliminary D.&C. is mandatory. The patient's capacity for being a few days pregnant at the time of such an operation is quite astonishing and can cause much subsequent embarrassment.

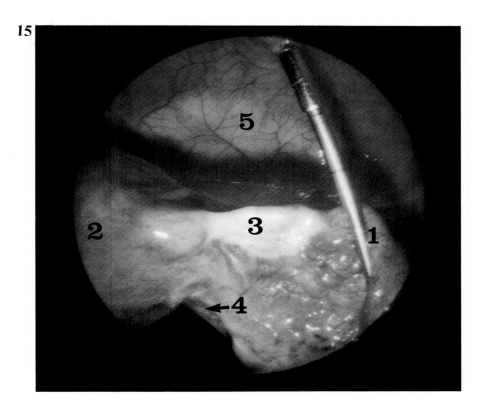

15 Diathermy of fallopian tube seen via laparoscope
A view seen through the laparoscope of the right fallopian tube after electrocautery. The tube is held laterally by the diathermy probe (1) and the various structures are numbered as follows: uterus (2), diathermised isthmal portion of tube (3), ovarian ligament (4), bladder (5).

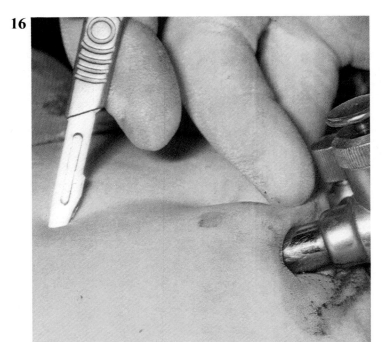 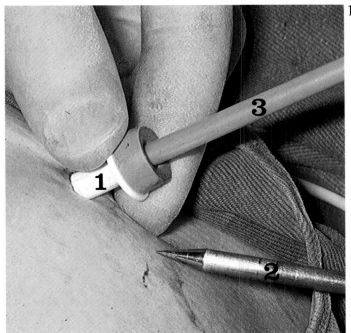

16 and 17 Introduction of diathermy electrode through second portal

The usual site of introduction of the diathermy electrode is lateral to the right rectus muscle 2.5 cm below the level of the umbilicus. The endoscope light is used to exclude the presence of blood vessels at the chosen site and a skin incision 1 cm long is made with the point of the scalpel as in Figure 16. The small trochar and cannula are inserted with due care in a slightly oblique direction medially and the cannula (1) is seen in position in Figure 17. The trochar (2) has been removed and the diathermy carrying rod (3) is introduced through the cannula. Both the cannula and the sheath of the diathermy electrode are insulated so that there should be no question of accidental burns of the abdominal wall.

In relation to accidental burns and when using diathermy intraperitoneally as in the following descriptions, it is wise to keep the diathermy electrode disconnected at all times other than when actually fulgurating the tube. The equipment may have an on-off switch; even so, a connected intraperitoneal diathermy point has the potential danger of a loaded gun and should be similarly regarded.

18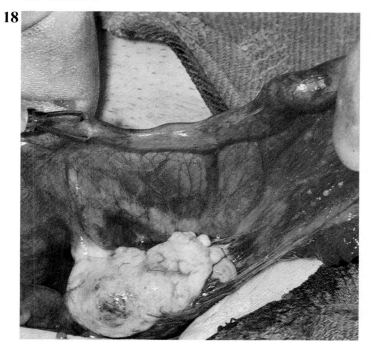

19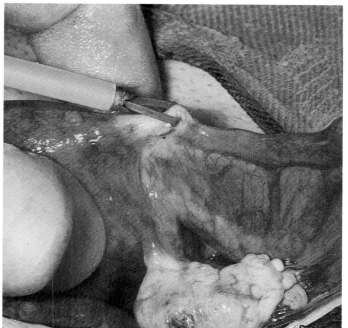

18 to 21 Diathermy sterilisation procedure (shown extra-abdominally for demonstration purposes)

In grasping the tube with the diathermy forceps in Figure 18 the hooks pick up the actual tube and not the mesosalpinx, otherwise the mesosalpinx will be fulgurated and the encircled tube largely escapes. The whitened burnt area is seen in Figure

19. The forceps are reapplied in Figure 20 at a distance of 1.5 cm and the treatment is repeated, causing a further area of blanching. The same procedure is repeated on the other tube and Figure 22 shows the diathermised tubes at the end of the

20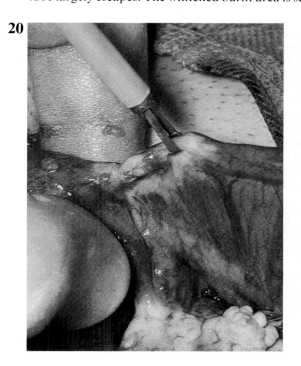

21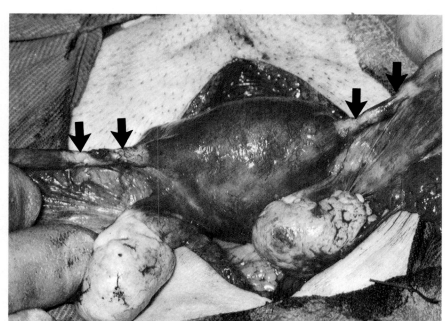

operation. The two points of electrocoagulation are arrowed.

Because the prospects of reversing diathermy sterilisation by tubal anastomosis are poor, and recognising that there will be occasional demands for reversal, the authors fulgurate the medial part of the tube so that there is sufficient viable tube left to implant into the uterus if required.

Non-diathermy methods of laparoscopic sterilisation

Silastic rings (Falope ring of elasticated silicone)

This method is attractive because no heat is required. The rings are applied to a small area of the tube. There is little damage to tissue and there is the advantage that reversal operations if required should be considerably easier. There are several drawbacks. Postoperative pain is sometimes severe immediately or for several weeks. There are reports of rings coming off the tube and it is possible to tear the tube with the forceps when applying them.

22 and 23 Equipment for tubal ring application

The necessary equipment is shown in Figure 22 and consists of a trochar (1) and cannula (2) for introduction of the ring applicator (3). Under magnification in Figure 23 the point of the applicator is seen to carry a Falope ring (4) ready for application and transferred to it by means of a metal cone-shaped attachment (5). It is pushed down on to the latter metal cone with the aid of the plastic pusher or handle (6) in the direction of the arrows.

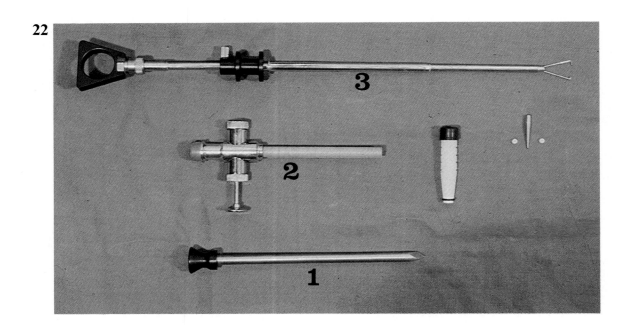

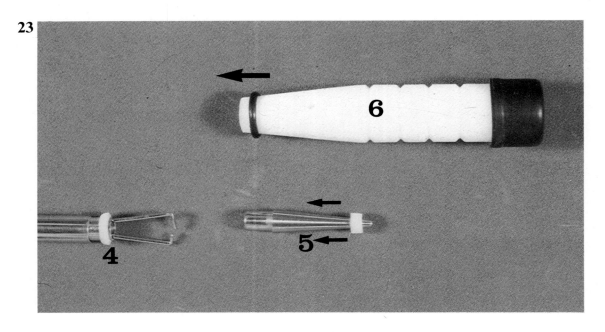

24 to 27 Application of Falope rings

The method is illustrated in Figures 24, 25 and 26 and is self explanatory. An important point is not to pull the tube away with the hooks before or during the application of the rings, otherwise division of the tube may result. There is a good loop of tube beyond the encircling ring; even so it appears that they do sometimes come off. Figure 27 shows the appearances after six months.

24

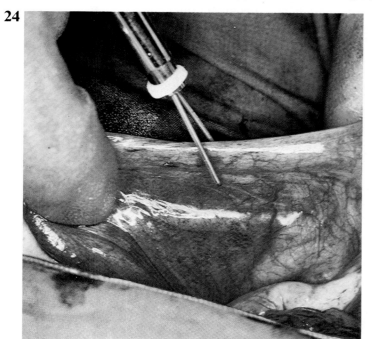

25

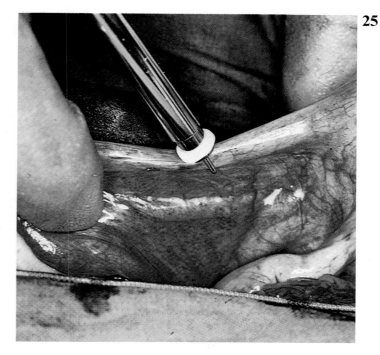

26

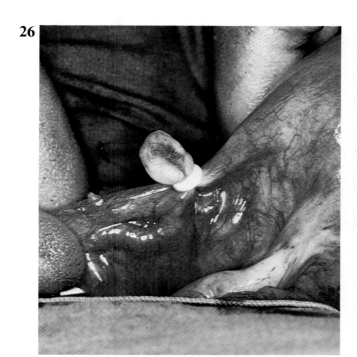

27

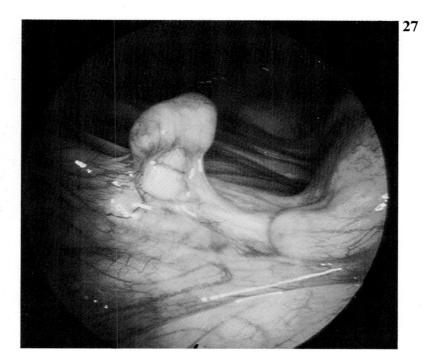

28

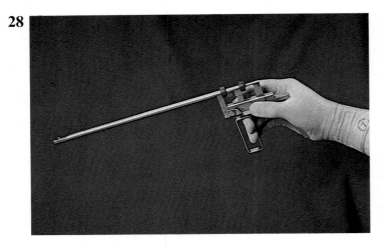

29

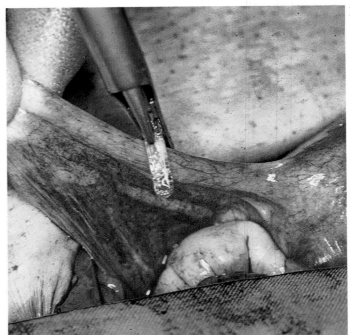

Spring-loaded clips (Hulka clips)

There are several types of clips but they are all made of plastic and the jaws are closed on the tube by means of an activating 'gun' or applicator. They are claimed to be very effective and the low failure rate is blamed on the restricted view through the laparoscope. Therefore, double portal application is advised in their placement. It has been claimed that if removed

30

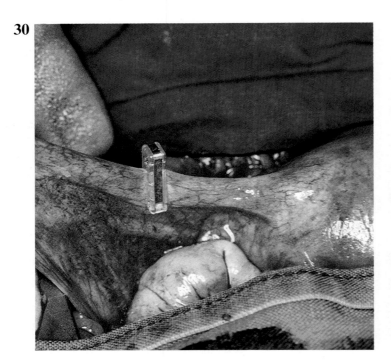

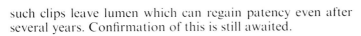

31

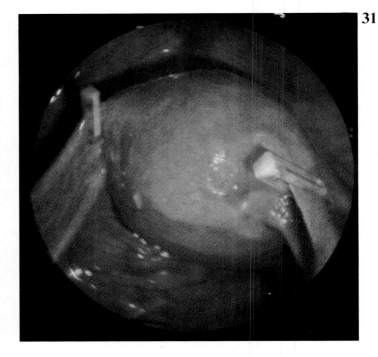

such clips leave lumen which can regain patency even after several years. Confirmation of this is still awaited.

28 Applicator for Hulka clips

Introduced in the same way the illustrated applicator or *'gun' is spring-loaded and having positioned the tube between the jaws of the actual clip, it is activated to close the clip on the tube.

*The appliance shown is from the Samaritan Hospital, London (by courtesy of Mr Brian Lieberman).

29 to 31 Application of Hulka clips

The method of approaching the tube is shown in Figure 29 and in Figure 30 the clip is in place. Figure 31 shows a laparoscopic view of the clips in position.

10: Cystourethropexy

Marshall–Marchetti–Krantz operation

The difficult problem of surgical treatment for genuine stress incontinence is referred to in Volume 1 of the Atlas. The authors state an unequivocal preference for the cruciate sling operation which they describe. Cystourethropexy, however, and especially the Marshall–Marchetti–Krantz operation, has a large following, both when vaginoplasty has already failed to cure stress incontinence and also as a primary procedure for the symptom when hysterectomy is being done in any case. The published results of the operation in many series are only moderate; in the opinion of the authors its worst feature is its lack of permanence. Despite some misgivings about its efficiency, the operation is illustrated and described because in some parts of the world it is looked on as the best prospect for cure of stress incontinence and no doubt will continue to be used in the forseeable future. The operation is not difficult to perform, but there are several possible snags that can lead to complications and have to be avoided. Technique has to be exact and that is taken into account and referred to in the text.

The principles of the operation are to open up the cave of Retzius and define the upper urethra and urethrovesical junction from above. This may be done after laparotomy or as a primary procedure and either a transverse or vertical incision is used. A No. 22 Foley catheter is *in situ* to outline the urethra and indicate the neck of the bladder. Paraurethral stitches are inserted in three equidistant pairs with one of each pair on the opposite side of the urethra from the other. These are subsequently stitched in the same progression to the periosteum of the posterior aspect of the pubic bone and thereby elevate the bladder neck and urethra to a new position. Postoperatively the bladder and urethra assume the general appearance seen in Diagram 1.

Because of the dangers to the bladder and urethra of the suspensory stitches, Burch and Barter both prefer to hitch up the lateral vaginal fornices to the ileopectineal line, but the principle is exactly the same. Chromicised catgut was originally advised for the supporting stitches but unabsorbable sutures are now more generally employed.

Stage 1: Exposure of upper urethra and bladder neck

1 Exposure of bladder retropubically

Whether or not laparotomy has been done, the peritoneum of the lower abdomen is retracted up and in a cephalad direction from the region of the symphysis pubis (1) to reveal the cave of Retzius and the fat surrounding the upper anterior surface of the bladder (2). The fingers can just be seen holding back the peritoneum with a gauze swab in the direction of the arrow (3) and the curved scissors are used to indicate the anterior aspect of the bladder.

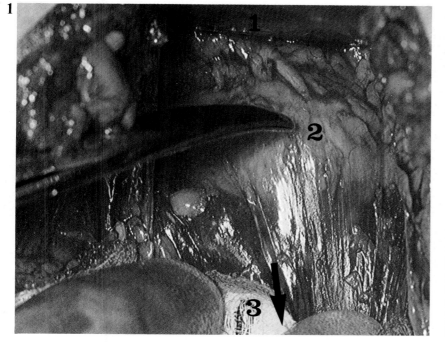

Position of bladder and urethra postoperatively

Structures numbered are: symphysis pubis (1), bladder (2), uterus (3), urethrovesical junction (4), paraurethral sutures (5).

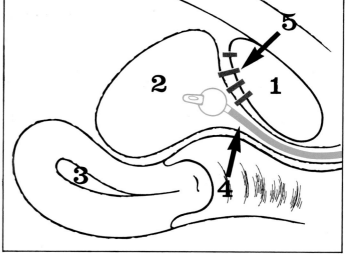

2

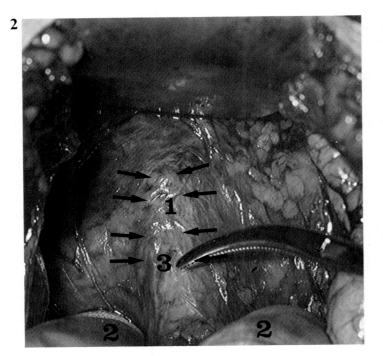

2 Bladder retracted to expose urethra

The fatty tissue has been swept laterally to expose the urethra (1) which has been further defined and dissected medially and which is outlined. The fingers (2) retain the bulb of the Foley catheter and the point of the curved forceps indicates the approximate position of the urethrovesical junction (3).

4

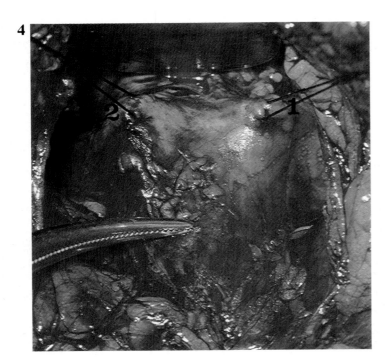

3

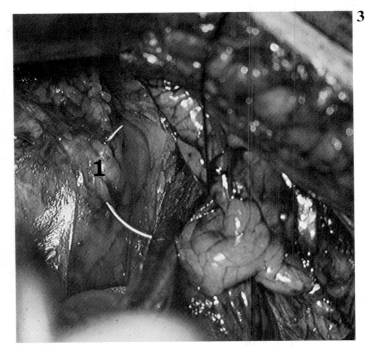

Stage 2: Placement of paraurethral suspension sutures

3 and 4 Placing distal paraurethral sutures

In Figure 3 the fine round-bodied needle carrying a No. 1 non-absorbable suture takes a firm bite which includes vaginal tissue lateral to the urethra on the right side and in the line of its axis (1). The urethra is easily palpable as it contains the No. 22 Foley catheter and the stitch is placed as far down the urethra as possible. In Figure 4 the matching stitch on the left side has also been placed (2) and the point of the forceps indicates the level of the urethrovesical angle as shown by the Foley catheter bulb.

5

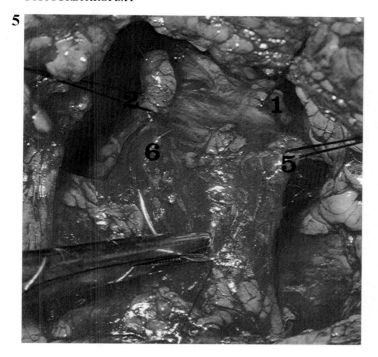

6

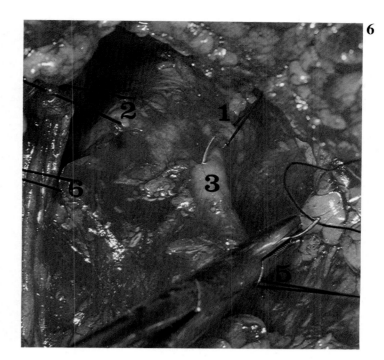

7

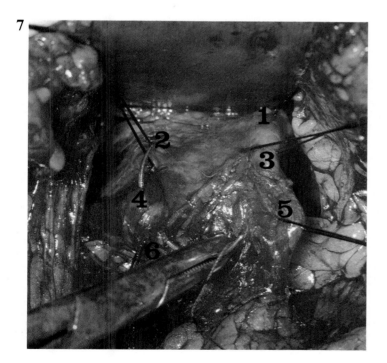

5 to 7 Placing proximal and intermediate pairs of paraurethral sutures

The proximal pair of sutures should be at the level of the bladder neck as indicated by the Foley catheter bulb and in Figure 5 that on the right has already been placed (5) and the left is being inserted (6). In Figure 6 an intermediate stitch (3) is being placed midway between (1) and (5) and in Figure 7 a matching intermediate stitch (4) midway between (2) and (6).

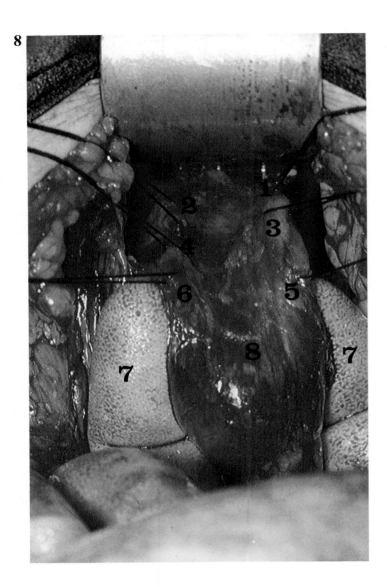

8 Paraurethral sutures in place

In this photograph the fingers (7) and (7) retract the bulb of the Foley catheter at the bladder neck (8) to display the two rows of paraurethral stitches (1), (3) and (5) on the right and matched by (2), (4) and (6) on the left.

Stage 3: Attaching sutures to retropubic periosteum

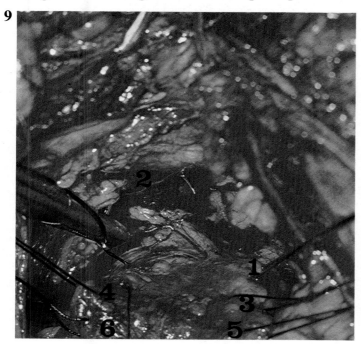

9 and 10 Attaching urethra and bladder neck to pubis (1)

In Figure 9 the needle carrying the left-sided distal suture (2) transfixes the periosteum of the pubis as shown. A round-bodied needle is used so as not to traumatise the bone. The other sutures are numbered as previously. In Figure 10 the same procedure is carried out on the right side with suture No. 1. Suture No. 2 is still untied.

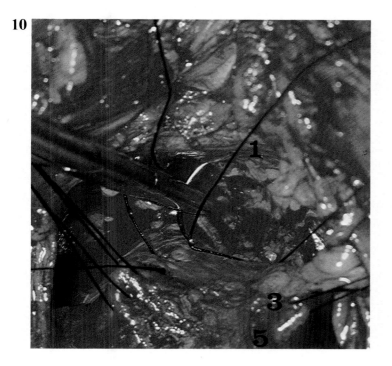

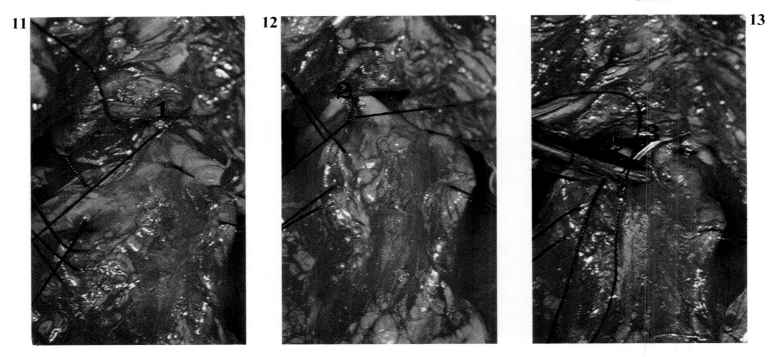

11 to 16 Attaching urethra and bladder neck to pubis (2)

In Figure 11 distal suture No. 1 is being tied and brings the urethra up close to the pubis. In Figure 12 suture No. 2 is being tied in the same way. In Figure 13 the intermediate suture No. 3 is taken through the periosteum on the needle and similarly with suture No. 4 in Figure 14. Suture No. 4 is being tied in Figure 15 and No. 3 tied in Figure 16.

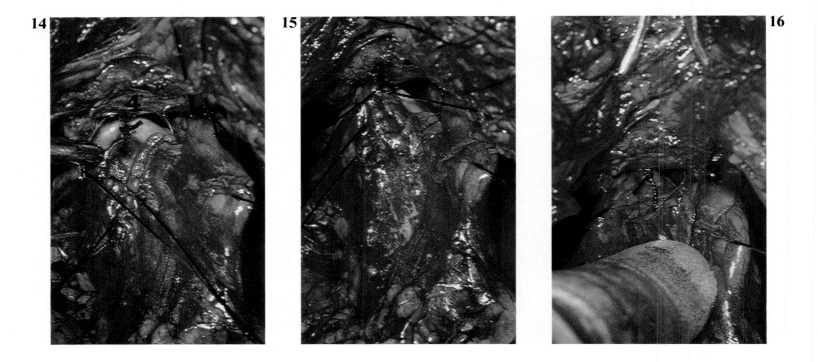

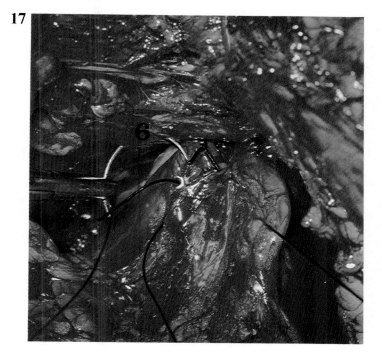

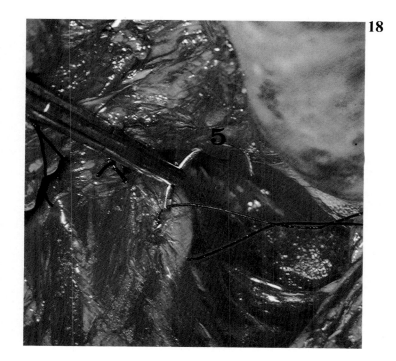

17 to 20 Attaching urethra and bladder neck to pubis (3)

The proximal sutures (No. 6 and 5) are similarly attached in Figures 17, 18, 19 and 20.

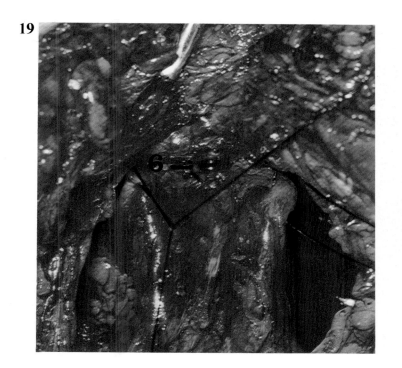

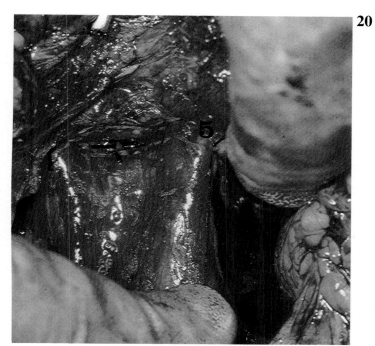

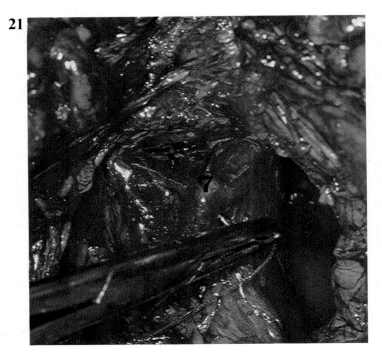

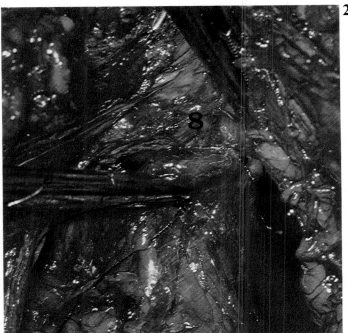

21 to 24 Attaching urethra and bladder neck to pubis (4)

It is considered important to insert further sutures to support the bladder neck in the midline by attaching the muscle wall of the upper aspect of the urethrovesical junction to the perichondrium of the symphysis pubis and the steps are shown. In Figure 21 the urethrovesical muscle is transfixed (7) and in Figure 22 the pericondrium is similarly transfixed (8) just lateral to the symphysis. The same is done on the other side (9 and 10) in Figures 23 and 24 respectively and the sutures tied. The bladder is now well hitched up retropubically and it only remains to close the abdomen. Drainage should not be necessary.

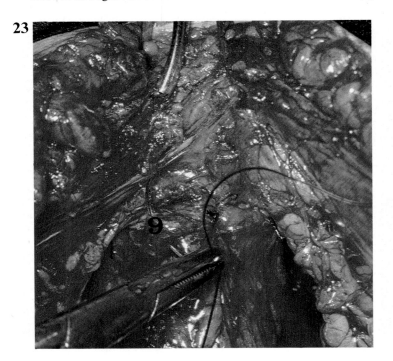

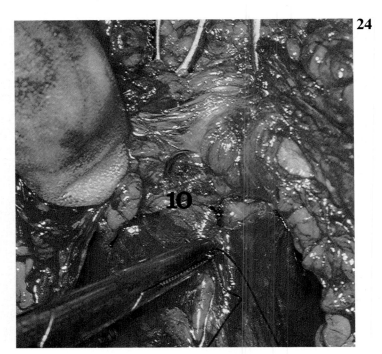

Stage 4: Obliteration of pouch of Douglas

It is claimed by some that there is a likelihood of enterocoele and vault prolapse developing as a result of the considerable advancement and displacement of the bladder and that in hysterectomy cases the pouch of Douglas should be closed; if this is so, and it seems logical to expect it, it emphasises still another unphysiological effect of the operation. There is already distortion of the bladder neck and upper urethra and in addition to that, the whole vaginal vault is displaced and held forward by the paraurethral sutures. There is evidence that this is not permanent, but it is inherent in the operation and the vault weakness should be allowed for.

The vaginal vault is supported in the following manner.

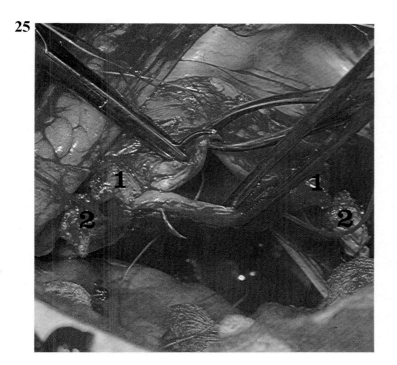

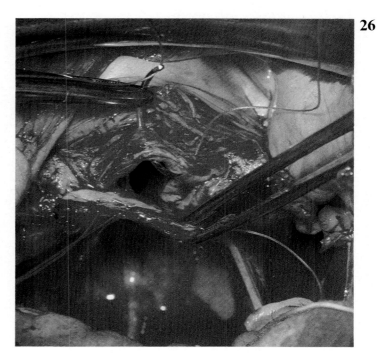

25 and 26 Closure of vaginal vault to incorporate uterosacral ligaments

In Figure 25 the lateral angles have been secured (1) and (1) and the ligated uterosacral ligaments are seen (2) and (2). The needle is completing the placement of a mattress suture towards the left side of the vault. In Figure 26 the same procedure is carried out on the right side. As each of these mattress sutures is tied it encircles and incorporates the uterosacral pedicle of its own side.

27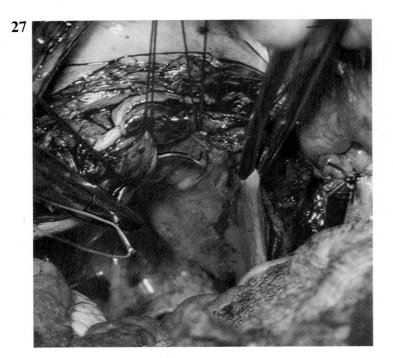

28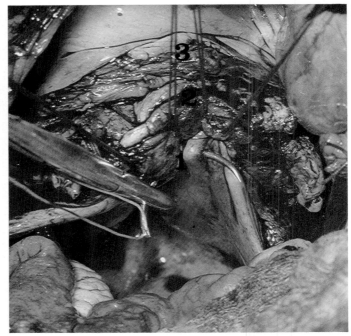

29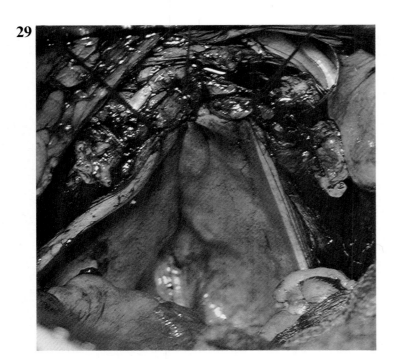

27 and 28 Obliteration of pouch of Douglas (1)

This is done by stitching the uterosacral ligaments together. The first stitch picks up the left ligament in Figure 27 and the right ligament in Figure 28. The various structures are numbered thus: uterosacral ligaments united (1), closed vaginal vault (2), and bladder (3).

29 Obliteration of pouch of Douglas (2)

Two stitches are already in place; three are usually sufficient.

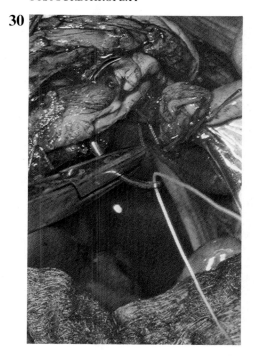

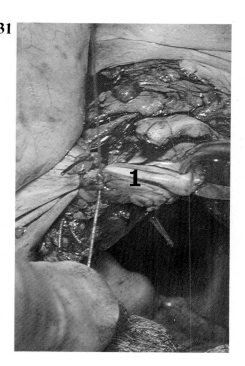

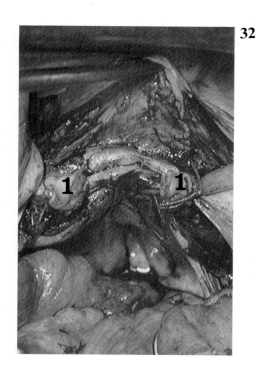

30 to 32 Fixing round ligaments to vault of vagina

As a possible aid to vault support the round ligaments are brought in and anchored to the vault. An anchor stitch is taken on the left side in Figure 30 and the left round ligament (1) drawn in and tied within it in Figure 31. Figure 32 shows both ligaments attached.

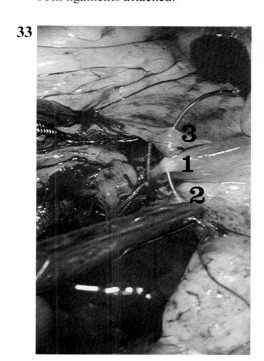

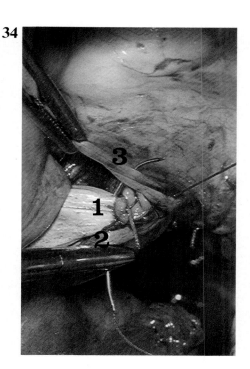

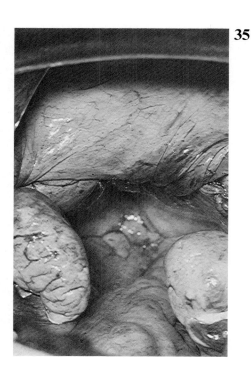

33 to 35 Closure of peritoneum

With the round ligaments drawn medially the area to be closed is less than usual. In Figure 33 the commencing stitch transfixes the posterior layer of the peritoneum (2), the surface of the round ligament (1) and then the anterior layer (3). In Figure 34 the same structures are involved at the end of the stitch and in Figure 35 the closed pelvic peritoneum is shown.

11: Ligation of internal iliac artery

Ligation of the internal iliac artery is an essential step in exenteration operations; otherwise it is only occasionally required to control severe and continuing haemorrhage. Such haemorrhage may result from various causes, most of them unexpected. A stage is reached in the operation where the surgeon realises that normal haemostatic measures are not succeeding and that the bleeding must be controlled without delay. The operation is not difficult and is nearly always spectacularly successful even when done on one side. In the type of pelvic side wall venous bleeding referred to in Chapter 1 it will help very little, because the bleeding is venous and the tributaries are inaccessible. The problems of that type of bleeding will be referred to in Volume 3. In ligating the artery the fragile internal iliac vein is carefully avoided and any temptation to ligate it also must be resisted. Ligation of the internal iliac vessel or vessels has no apparent detrimental effect on the patient, although some textbooks warn against its use if heavy preoperative radiotherapy has been given. Number 2 catgut is generally used to tie the artery which is not itself divided.

The operation described is envisaged as an emergency measure. The aim should therefore be to secure the entire trunk easily and quickly with a view to turning off the blood flow. It can be dangerous and time consuming to seek the anterior branch only, although that may be surgically more correct. To do so risks danger to accompanying veins with more bleeding, so that the disadvantages quickly come to outweigh the advantages.

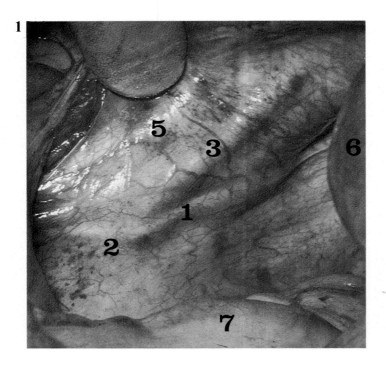

1 General view of iliac vessels and ureter (left)

The abdominal contents are held back by the fingers to demonstrate the anatomy at the pelvic brim. Through the peritoneum the outline of the ureter (1) is seen crossing the common iliac artery (2). The external iliac artery (3) is easily visible with the psoas muscle (5) lateral to it. The uterus is medial (6) and the rectum is in the foreground (7).

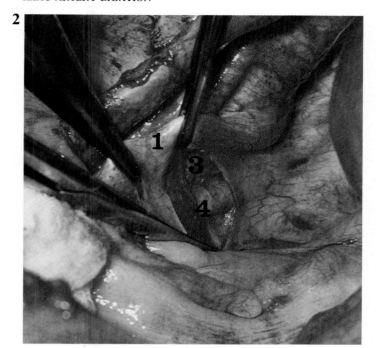

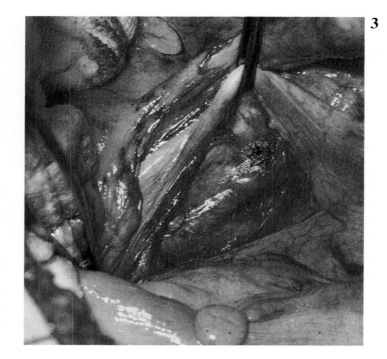

2 to 4 Exposure of left ureter

The peritoneum has been opened with the scissors in Figure 2 and the ureter (1) is lifted up to give a view of the external (3) and internal (4) iliac arteries. In Figure 3 dissection has progressed a stage further and in Figure 4 the internal iliac artery (4) is being lifted up on the points of the curved forceps.

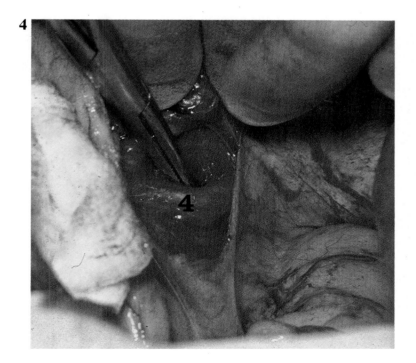

5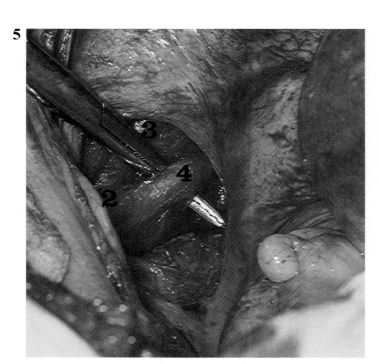

6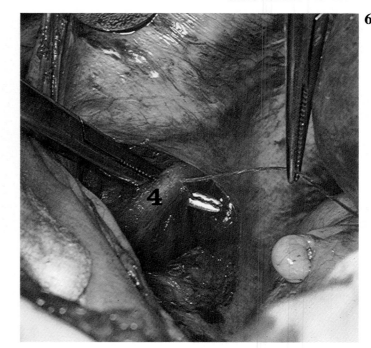

5 to 7 Ligation of internal iliac artery (left)

In Figure 5 the internal iliac artery (4) and the external iliac artery (3) are seen clearly just at the bifurcation of the common iliac artery (2). The forceps are under the internal iliac artery. In Figure 6 the ligature is picked up by the forceps and in Figure 7 it is ready to be tied.

7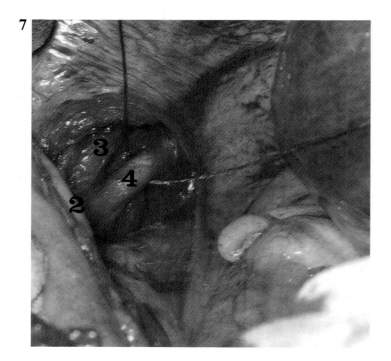

8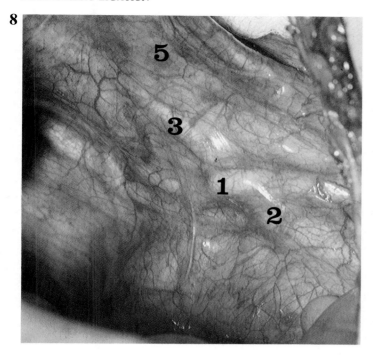

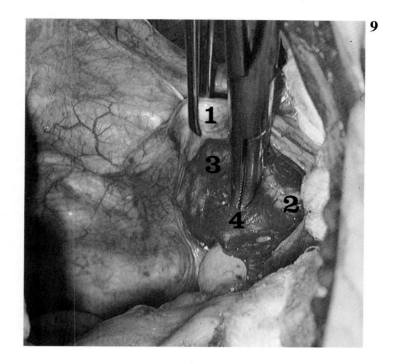 **9**

8 to 11 Ligation of internal artery (right)

The same points and procedures are shown on the right side with the structures numbered similarly. Ureter (1), common iliac artery (2), external iliac artery (3), internal iliac artery (4), psoas muscle (5).

10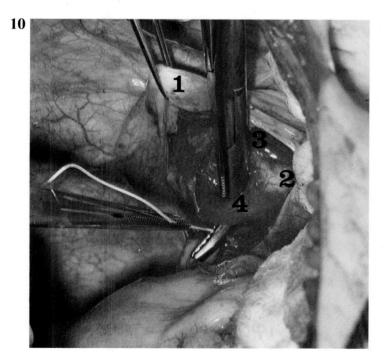

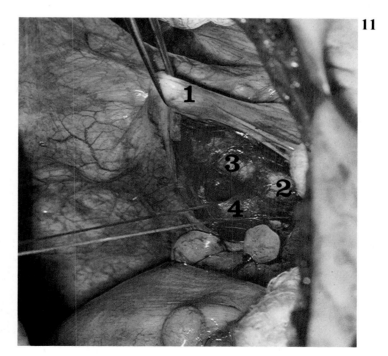 **11**

12: Drainage of abdominal wound haematoma

The most meticulous surgeon will be rewarded occasionally by the development of a postoperative haematoma in the abdominal wound. Haematomata are often the product of imprecise or hurried surgery but may sometimes result from reactionary haemorrhage, a minor blood-clotting defect or pre-existing infection at the operative site. From time to time a patient will subject her early postoperative wound to unreasonable strain and cause the tearing or freeing of a sealed off blood vessel. The usual site of haematomata is superficial to the rectus sheath and bleeding occurs into the loose fatty tissue. The wound looks swollen, is tender, and the patient is mildly pyrexial and not very well. If not dealt with the haematoma becomes infected and in due course discharges pus. Unless proper drainage is then instituted recovery is very slow and the wound becomes fibrotic and distorted.

At other times the haematoma is at a deeper level – between the rectus muscle and the anterior sheath or deep to the muscle and spreading extraperitoneally. In either case there is pain, pyrexia, tachycardia and a degree of ileus. Exploration of the wound is mandatory and relief immediate. The haematoma may take the form of a large extraperitoneal collection of blood or a restricted area of considerable tension underneath the aponeurosis. The management of a case typifying each variety is illustrated.

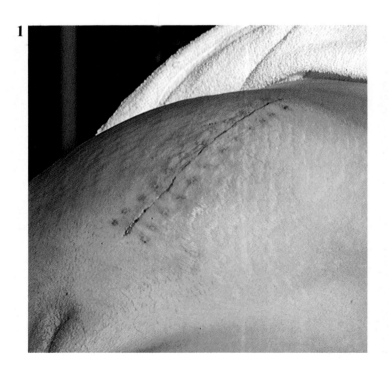

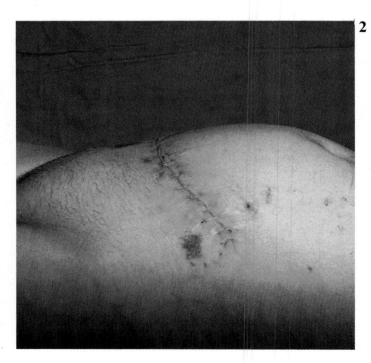

1 Superficial haematoma: preoperative appearance

The swollen, discoloured and fluctuant wound was seen at the sixth postoperative day. The patient was pyrexial and the haematoma was obviously infected. The condition should have been recognised and the contents evacuated earlier.

2 Deep haematoma: preoperative appearance

There is obvious bowel distention as well as local swelling above the wide transverse incision. The patient was at the fourth postoperative day after hysterectomy for widespread chronic pelvic infection. She had pyrexia, tachycardia, some degree of ileus and pain in the wound.

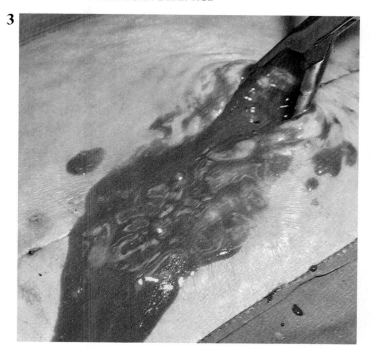

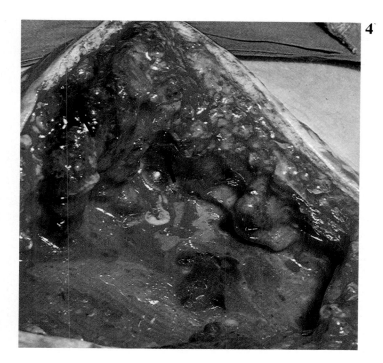

3 to 5 Opening superficial infected haematoma

Sinus forceps have been pushed through the scar and the limbs opened to allow the escape of a flood of stinking *E. coli* pus in Figure 3. Figure 4 shows the wound opened up in its length with pus still draining from it. Parts of the haematoma (arrowed) are still seen so that the source of the trouble is obvious. In Figure 5 the abscess cavity is empty and shows how the pus had undermined and distended the superficial fascia and skin. Pieces of haematoma are still visible (arrowed). The abdomen is viewed obliquely in these photographs. The symphysis pubis is to the left and the umbilicus to the right (1).

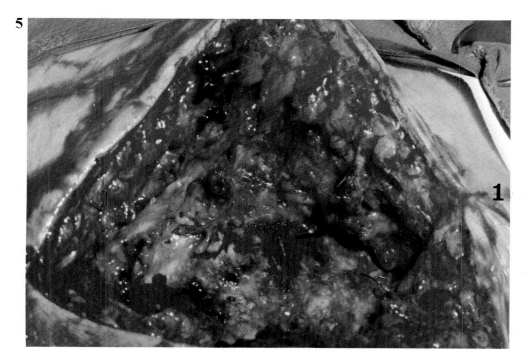

6

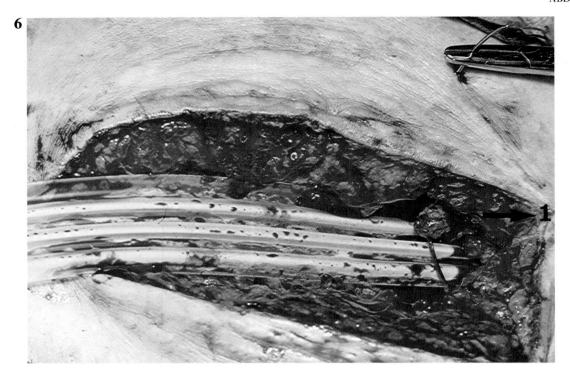

7

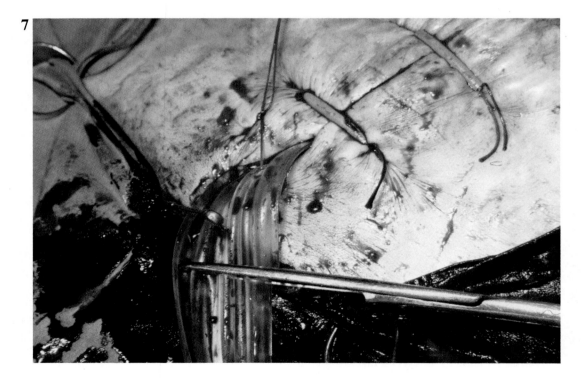

6 and 7 Drainage of superficial infected haematoma

In Figure 6 a wide corrugated plastic drain is laid along the floor of the abscess cavity on the rectus sheath and in the length of the wound. The umbilicus is on the right of the photograph (1). The first deep tension suture to approximate the full thickness of skin and superficial fascia has transfixed the right side and will complete its journey on the left. In Figure 7 the wound edges have been approximated without tension by rubber-covered full-thickness stitches as shown. The drain is fixed to the skin by a stitch and a safety pin has been attached, while the excess drain is cut off. Antibiotics are given and the drain removed in 48 hours. Recovery is rapid.

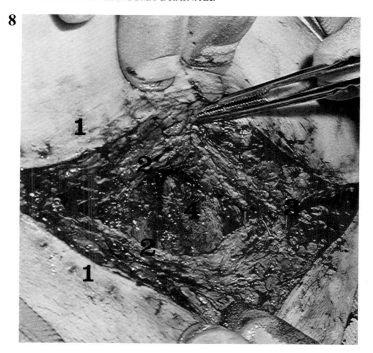

8 Exploration of deep wound haematoma (1)

The skin stitches (1) and (1) have been removed and the rectus sheath (2) and (2) is being opened. The sheath suture was intact and is seen being loosened at (3). The rectus muscle (4) looks healthy and there is no sign of haematoma or abscess at this level.

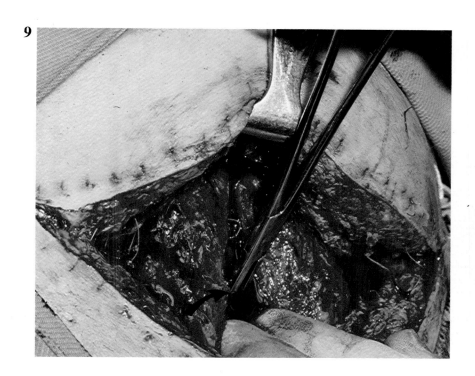

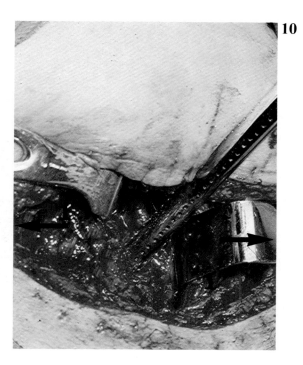

9 and 10 Exploration of deep wound haematoma (2)

In Figure 9 a forceps probing between the recti muscle discovers a haematoma of partially liquid and partially clotted blood on the deep surface of the muscles and lying extraperitoneally where arrowed. It is under moderate tension. In Figure 10 the recti muscles (1) and (1) are retracted laterally (in the direction of the arrows) and the sucker evacuates the haematoma as shown. There is no residual bleeding from the cavity.

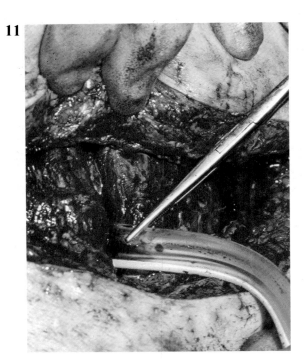

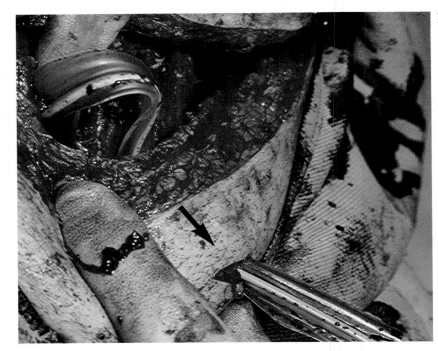

11 to 14 Drainage of deep wound haematoma

In Figure 11 a 2 cm wide strip of corrugated plastic drain is introduced into the haematoma cavity with sinus forceps and placed in its depth with the fingers. In Figure 12 an incision has been made below the wound and the end of the drain is being drawn through it so that drainage will be dependent. The upper end of the drain is held in the cavity meantime. In

Figure 13 the edges of the recti muscles are approximated gently with one or two fine sutures before closing the full thickness of the skin, superficial fascia, deep fascia and rectus sheath in one layer. Monofilmament nylon sutures are used and the course taken by the needle in placing the stitch is indicated. In Figure 14 the wound is seen closed by vertical mattress

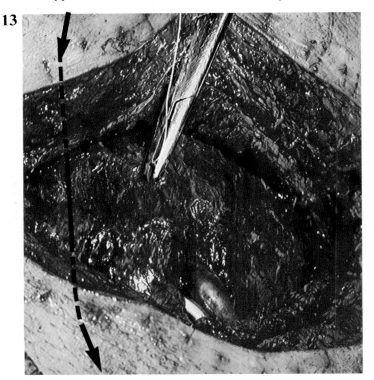

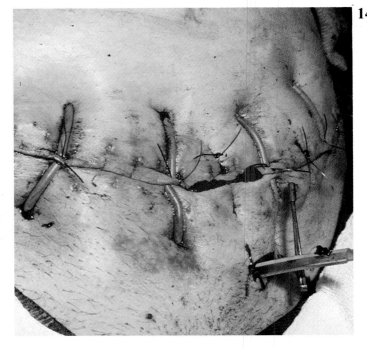

tension sutures which are rubber-sheathed to avoid cutting into the skin. The drain is fixed to the skin and has a safety pin attached for recognition. Postoperative management includes the giving of antibiotics; the drain is removed after 48 hours.

13: Abdominal closure of pelvic fistulae

Fistulae between the vagina and the urinary or alimentary tract necessarily demand closure, but this is not always easy and it is very important that the correct surgical approach be adopted. The two problems are considered separately.

Vesicovaginal or ureterovaginal fistulae

Generally, vesicovaginal fistulae are better dealt with vaginally and the principles of treatment are illustrated and described in Volume 1 of the Atlas. That such cases are sometimes very complex and not what they may seem was emphasised; that warning is repeated here. Vesicovaginal fistulae close to the ureteric orifices and all ureterovaginal fistulae must be dealt with abdominally. The operation may be done extravesically or transvesically or both but the peritoneal cavity is usually opened. The authors do not intend to become involved in a detailed description of what can be a very specialised form of urological surgery; but a case of a massive vesicovaginal fistula with ureteric involvement is illustrated because it incorporates nearly all the points of technique and shows what may be entailed in closure of a complex vesicovaginal fistula. The findings are represented diagramatically (Diagram 1).

The whole base of the bladder was missing, the right ureter was blocked and almost totally detached from the bladder at its lower end. There was right hydronephrosis and hydroureter with very little function in the right kidney. An extraperitoneal approach defined the dilated right ureter which had almost separated off from the bladder. The bladder vault was then approached transperitoneally and opened in the midline. After catheterising the left ureter the large basal fistula was excised and vagina and bladder closed separately and at right angles to each other. The detached right ureter was reimplanted into the bladder and the vault of the bladder subsequently closed around a drain. The details are shown and described in the text.

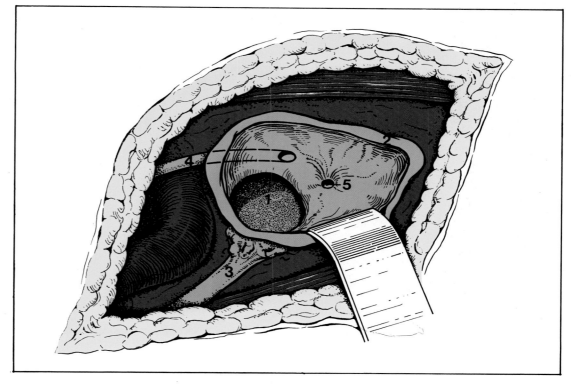

Diagram 1
Fistulous opening in bladder (1), bladder wall (2), right ureter (3) left ureter (4), internal urethral orifice (5).

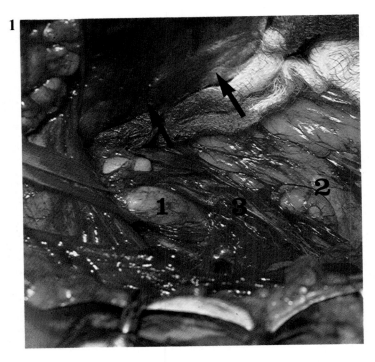

1 Exposure of right ureter extraperitoneally (1)

The distended right ureter (1) has been underrun with a tape and is being followed down towards the bladder (2) while the peritoneum and abdominal contents are pulled medially by the retractor in the direction of the arrows. The lower end of the ureter disappears into an area of amorphous tissue (3) which fell apart during blunt dissection and the ureter became detached completely from the bladder.

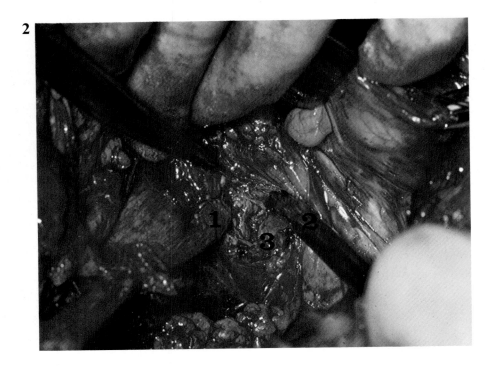

2 Exposure of right ureter extraperitoneally (2)

The end of the ureter (1) is seen free of the bladder and a catheter (2) has been introduced into the bladder at the site of the former ureteric attachment. Note the thickened tissue (3) and the ureter already less distended.

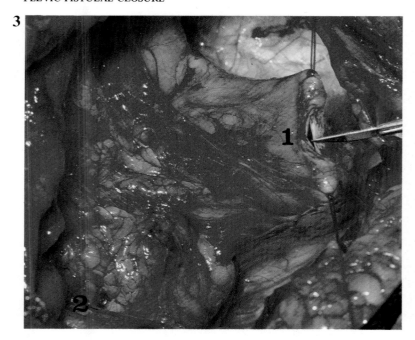

3 Opening vault of bladder

The peritoneal cavity has now been opened and after the insertion of two stay sutures, the bladder is opened in the midline on its upper surface (1). The site of the detached ureter with the catheter is just visible at (2).

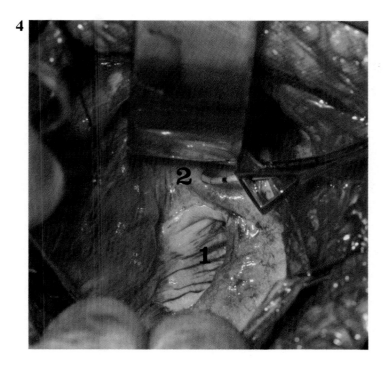

4 Bladder opened and left ureter catheterised

The bladder has now been opened on its upper surface and the huge vesicovaginal fistula is seen on its base (1). A catheter has been passed into the left ureter (2) for definition.

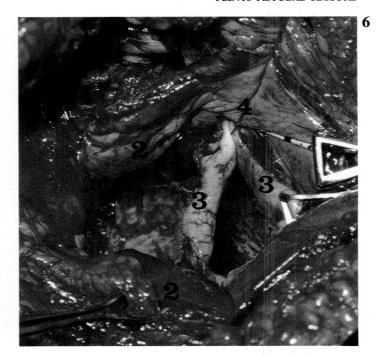

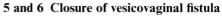

5 and 6 Closure of vesicovaginal fistula

The fibrous edge of the fistula is first excised to allow separate closure of vagina and bladder. The approach merits some explanation. It is transvesical but the bladder incision has been extended backwards to meet the fistula thus bisecting the bladder posteriorly. In Figure 5 the fistulous edge (1) is held in Littlewood's and dissecting forceps while it is excised quite widely with scissors. In Figure 6 the two halves of the bladder have retracted laterally (2) and (2) while the vaginal edge (3) is being closed transversely with interrupted PGA No. 1 sutures. A holding stitch has been inserted (4) and the edges will be everted towards the vagina by the sutures.

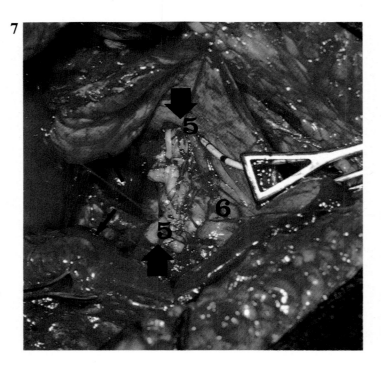

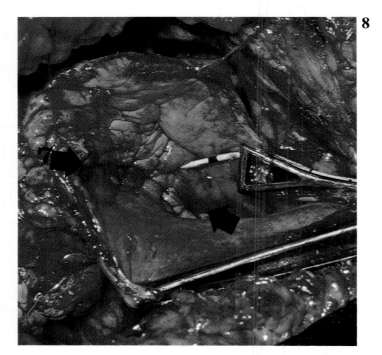

7 and 8 Completion of closure

The transverse closure is complete with the ends held up by sutures (5) and (5) while the first stitch in the anteroposterior closure of the bladder muscle has been inserted at (6). The arrows indicate the bladder edges to be approximated. The direction of the suture line is between the broad arrows. In Figure 8 the anteroposterior approximation of the bladder base has been completed with the bladder closed at right angles to the vagina. It is closed in two layers, the muscle layer with PGA No. 0 suture and then an inverted submucosal layer using No. 00 catgut. This last stitch is seen being tied off at (7) and the direction of the suture line is between the broad arrows.

9

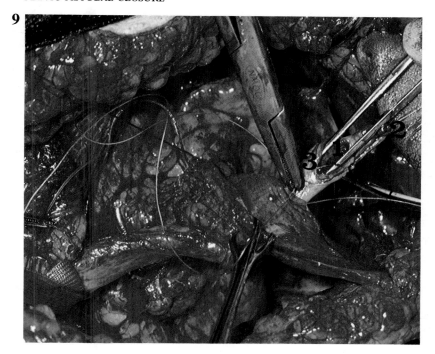

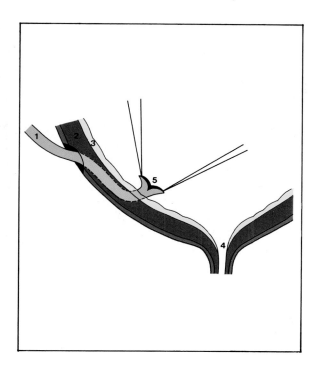

9 Reimplanting the right ureter into the bladder (i)

In Figure 9 the end of the ureter (1) has been split in fish-mouth fashion. It is drawn into the bladder along a track or tunnel made by forceps which pierce the muscle wall and then run submucosally for a distance before piercing the bladder wall; this is indicated in Diagram 2. This technique ensures a better blood supply to the ureter with less scarring and prevents urine reflux. The sutures on the fish-mouth end are numbered (2) and (3) with the latter shown being inserted.

Diagram 2
1 Ureter
2 Smooth muscle
3 Mucosa
4 Internal urethral orifice
5 Split end of ureter ready to be stitched to bladder mucosa

10

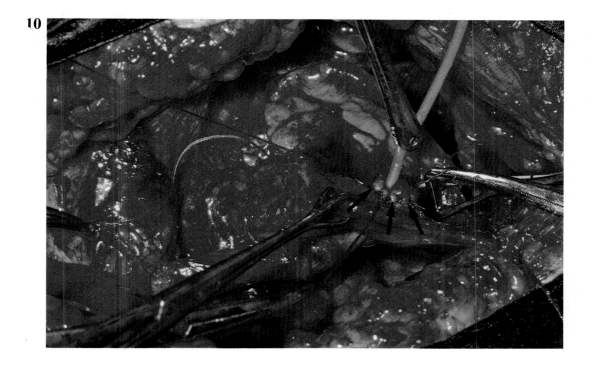

10 Reimplanting the right ureter into the bladder (ii)

The open ends of the ureter are stitched to the bladder musosa by the holding sutures and any necessary additional ones (arrowed). A ureteric catheter is inserted for support and drainage postoperatively and will subsequently drain per urethram.

11
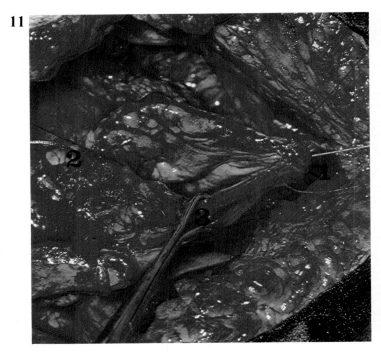

12
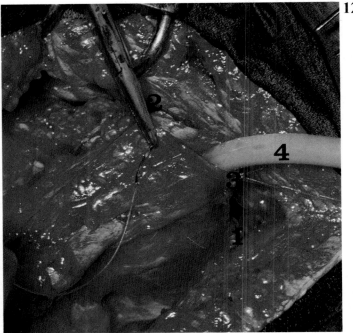

11 to 13 Closure of vault of bladder: muscle layer

The bladder is now closed in two layers with a Foley catheter at the midpoint of the suture line for additional drainage suprapubically. In Figure 11 a continuous muscle stitch is commencing anteriorly (1) while the posterior limit of the bladder vault (2) is held taut, and the right edge pulled back by tissue forceps (3) at the midpoint. In Figure 12 the catheter (4) is in place with the anterior half of the vault already closed between numbers (1) and (3) and commencing closure of the other half between numbers (2) and (3). Figure 13 shows the vault of the bladder completely closed.

13
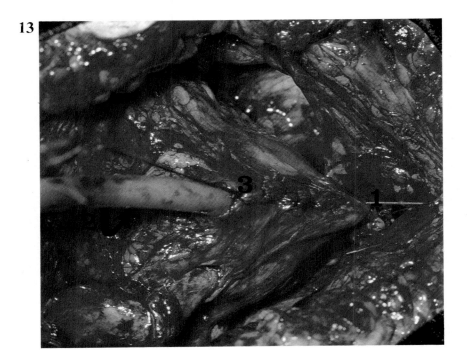

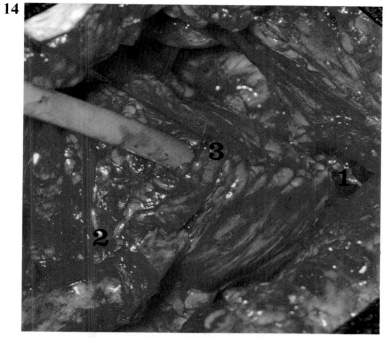

14 Closure of vault of bladder complete

This illustration shows the vault closure more clearly as an apparently curving line between the anterior (1) and the posterior (2) ends of the bladder vault incision. The stitch is still uncut at the mid-point (3) with the Foley catheter adjacent to it. The muscle closure has been reinforced by a Lembert suture on the visceral peritoneum of the bladder so that there is no raw area.

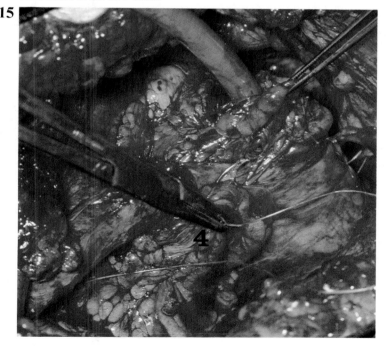

15 Supporting stitches for implanted ureter

Redundant paravesical tissue is picked up by a fine stitch (4) and used to cover and reinforce the ureter at the site of implantation.

Rectovaginal or enterovaginal fistulae

Fistulae situated low in the vagina or near the introitus can be closed from below; the technique is described in Volume 4 of the Atlas. Apart from these, practically all other enterovaginal and some rectovaginal fistulae need to be closed by the abdominal route. The reason is that there is a fistulous track of varying length between the two cavities and this needs to be defined, separated and the defect in the bowel wall surgically closed. More often than not and because there has been an underlying condition such as diverticulitis, the distorted and affected part of the bowel involved in the fistula has to be resected. Having established that a rectovaginal fistula is not amenable to closure from below, most gynaecologists pass the case to an abdominal surgeon as was in fact done here. The case is briefly described because the preliminary investigations and the decision as to how it should be managed both fell within the sphere of the gynaecologist.

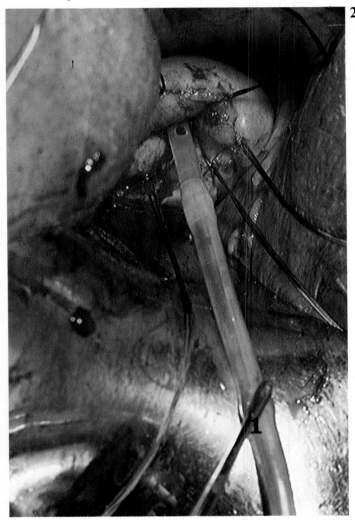

In the operation it was established that the fistulous track between the vagina and the sigmoid colon was of considerable length. On laparotomy the affected coil of bowel was identified and the fistula separated from the vaginal wall which was then closed. The area of the sigmoid colon was the site of diverticulitis and was resected. The principal details are illustrated and described in the text.

1 Exploration of fistulous track

A medium-sized uterine dilator is used to explore the track of the fistula. The vaginal wall surrounding the fistula is steadied by a series of holding sutures while the cervix is pulled up and hidden by the upper vaginal retractor.

2 Estimating length of vaginointestinal track

A Foley catheter has been passed along the track of the fistula into the lumen of the bowel and the bulb inflated. The catheter is then held back against the bowel wall by pulling on the vaginal end and the distance of the bowel cavity from the vagina is measured on the catheter. The distance is indicated by the sinus forceps on the catheter (1) and after the removal of the catheter the actual length can be measured: in this case 5 cm. Another method of measuring the length and showing the direction of the track is by sialography.

3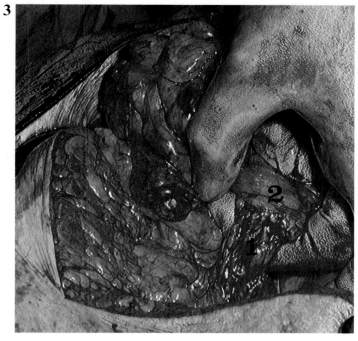

4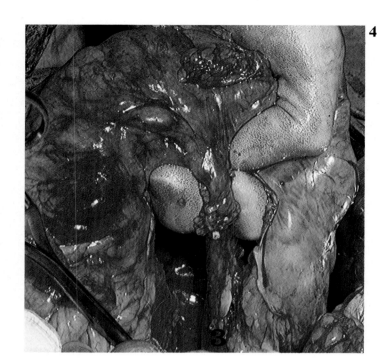

3 and 4 Defining fistulous track abdominally

At laparotomy the track (1) was found to run from the sigmoid colon (2) to the vaginal wall (3). The upper end is seen hooked on the finger in Figure 3 and in Figure 4 the track has been dissected clear of surrounding structures.

5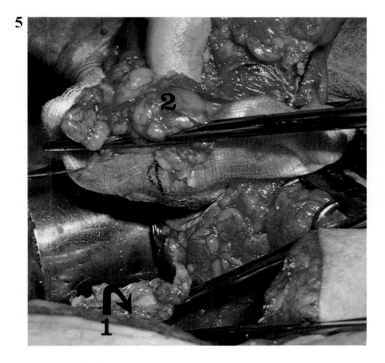

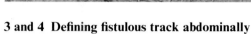

6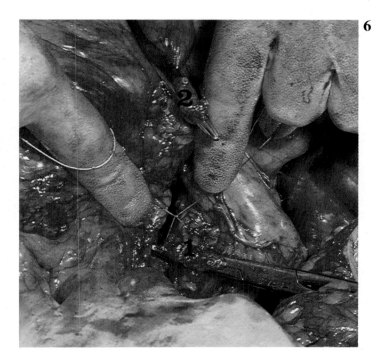

5 and 6 Division and ligation of vaginal end of fistula

The vaginal end of the track is deep in the pelvis and has been cut across with scissors in Figure 5 at (1) while the upper end is free at (2). The vaginal end has been transfixed and is being ligated with PGA No. 1 suture in Figure 6.

7

8

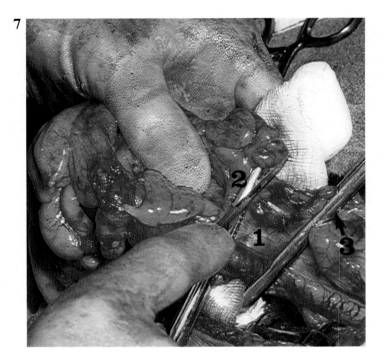

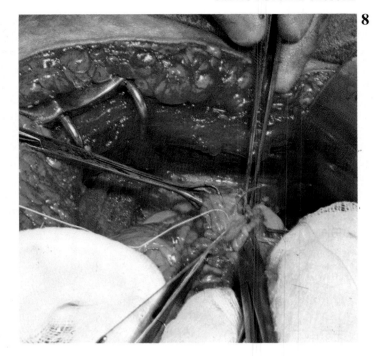

7 and 8 Resection of affected loop of bowel

It was considered necessary to excise the loop of sigmoid colon which included the intestinal end of the fistula; in Figure 7 the bowel (1) is seen being divided between a crushing (2) and an anastomotic (3) clamp. In Figure 8 end-to-end anastomosis of the bowel is in progress after resection of the affected loop.

Index

Index

Index

Contents of further volumes in the Gynaecological Surgery series

Volume 1: Vaginal Operations

1 **Dilatation and Curettage**

2 **Diathermy Coagulation of the Cervix**

3 **Cryosurgical Treatment of Cervical Erosion**

4 **Removal of Sub-mucus Fibroid Polyp**
   Vaginal excision

5 **Manchester Repair**
   Anterior and posterior wall repair

6 **Repair of Enterocele**

7 **Repair of Rectocele**

8 **Vaginal Hysterectomy**

9 **Post-Hysterectomy Prolapse**

10 **Surgical Treatment of Stress Incontinence**
   Cruciate bladder sling technique

11 **Vaginoplasty**
   Repair of localised vaginal constriction

12 **Repair of Vesico-Vaginal Fistula**

Volume 3: Operations For Malignant Disease

Volume 4: Surgery Of Vulva And Lower Genital Tract

Volume 5: Infertility Surgery

1 **Instruments and Developmental Anatomy**

2 **Preliminary Investigations**
  Hysterosalpingography
  Intrauterine aspiration curettage (Vabra)
  Laparoscopy

3 **Cervical Operations**
  Trachelorraphy
  Cervical cerclage (Shirodkar operation)

4 **Utero-Vaginal Operations for Congenital Malformations**
  Division of vaginal septum
  Uteroplasty (Strassman's operation)

5 **Tubo-Ovarian Operations**
  Salpingolysis
  Salpingostomy
  Salpingostomy with prostheses
  Implantation of Fallopian tube
  Fallopian tubal reanastomosis
  Conservative surgery of pelvic endometriosis

6 **Microsurgical Techniques in Infertility Surgery**
  Implantation and reanastomosis of Fallopian tubes

Volume 6: Surgery Of Conditions Complicating Pregnancy

1 **Instruments and Surgical Anatomy in Pregnancy**

2 **Evacuation of Uterus**
   Incomplete miscarriage
   Hydatidiform mole

3 **Termination of Pregnancy**
   During first trimester (suction curettage)
   Under local anaesthetic (Karman cannula)
   During second trimester (intra and extra amniotic drug instillation)

4 *Abdominal Hysterotomy*

5 *Cervical Cerclage (Shirodkar operation)*

6 *Ovarian Cyst in Pregnancy*

7 *Appendicectomy in Pregnancy*

8 **Ectopic Pregnancy Surgery**
   For complete tubal rupture (salpingectomy)
   For intratubal haematocele (tubal conservation)
   For abdominal pregnancy

9 *Caesarean Section (Lower Segment)*

10 *Surgical Management of Uterine Choriocarcinoma*
   (gestational trophoblastic disease)